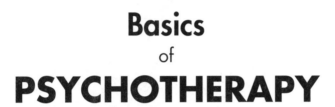

Basics

of

PSYCHOTHERAPY

A Practical Guide to
Improving Clinical Success

Basics
of
PSYCHOTHERAPY

A Practical Guide to
Improving Clinical Success

by

Richard B. Makover, M.D.

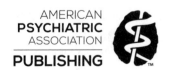
AMERICAN
PSYCHIATRIC
ASSOCIATION

PUBLISHING

Note: The authors have worked to ensure that all information in this book is accurate at the time of publication and consistent with general psychiatric and medical standards, and that information concerning drug dosages, schedules, and routes of administration is accurate at the time of publication and consistent with standards set by the U.S. Food and Drug Administration and the general medical community. As medical research and practice continue to advance, however, therapeutic standards may change. Moreover, specific situations may require a specific therapeutic response not included in this book. For these reasons and because human and mechanical errors sometimes occur, we recommend that readers follow the advice of physicians directly involved in their care or the care of a member of their family.

Books published by American Psychiatric Association Publishing represent the findings, conclusions, and views of the individual authors and do not necessarily represent the policies and opinions of American Psychiatric Association Publishing or the American Psychiatric Association.

If you wish to buy 50 or more copies of the same title, please go to www.appi.org/specialdiscounts for more information.

Copyright © 2017 Richard B. Makover, M.D.
ALL RIGHTS RESERVED

Manufactured in the United States of America on acid-free paper
21   20   19   18   17   5   4   3   2   1
First Edition

Typeset in Palatino Light Standard and Futura Standard Book.

American Psychiatric Association Publishing
A Division of American Psychiatric Association
1000 Wilson Boulevard
Arlington, VA 22209–3901
www.appi.org

Library of Congress Cataloging-in-Publication Data
Names: Makover, Richard B., author.
Title: Basics of psychotherapy : a practical guide to improving clinical success / by Richard B. Makover.
Description: First edition. | Arlington, Virginia : American Psychiatric Association Publishing, [2017] | Includes bibliographical references and index.
Identifiers: LCCN 2017004882 (print) | LCCN 2017005674 (ebook) | ISBN 9781615370764 (pbk. : alk. paper) | ISBN 9781615371327 (ebook)
Subjects: | MESH: Psychotherapy--methods | Psychological Theory
Classification: LCC RC480 (print) | LCC RC480 (ebook) | NLM WM   420 | DDC 616.89/14—dc23
LC record available at https://lccn.loc.gov/2017004882

British Library Cataloguing in Publication Data
A CIP record is available from the British Library.

To my patients and my supervisors:
I learned from all of them

CONTENTS

Preface

Over the course of a long career, I have had the opportunity to observe other professionals practice a variety of psychotherapies. They demonstrated a wide spectrum of skills. Certain clinicians showed great competence and expertise in their work with patients, and I was fortunate to learn from them both by their example and by their guidance. Others, while diligent and conscientious, were not as effective. Some practitioners struggled with certain kinds of cases and succeeded with others. Some appeared to form strong bonds with their patients, but their results were disappointing: patients dropped out of treatment or continued for long periods without significant improvement. Whether these therapists were new to practice or quite experienced, I observed that these difficulties often seemed to reflect an incomplete grounding in the basic principles of psychotherapy.

Doing therapy well is difficult. A strong foundation in the universal principles of therapeutic practice can improve patient outcomes while helping to manage inherent challenges such as clinician stress, fatigue, and burnout. I have found, however, that these core principles may not be fully covered in the coursework, training, or supervision offered by many professional programs.

My intent in this book is to provide a practical guide to the essential postulates and practices that form the foundation of successful treatment. These principles are not specific to any one type of therapy, but rather form the basis of effective therapeutic work regardless of the specific methodological approach. This book is addressed to those therapists who are open to reexamining the essential elements of their craft and applying these elements directly to their everyday work. My belief is that therapists who expand their understanding of these ideas and practices will gain in confidence and expertise, improve patient outcomes, and increase their personal satisfaction with the art of psychotherapy.

About the Author

Richard B. Makover was educated at Yale University and the Albert Einstein College of Medicine. After a medical internship, he completed his psychiatric training as chief resident, served two years as a U.S. Navy psychiatrist, and opened a private psychiatric practice. His knowledge of psychiatry is based on more than 40 years of clinical experience in office-based, ambulatory, and inpatient settings. Dr. Makover has held academic positions at Cornell University Medical College and The New York Medical College. He is a Lecturer at the Yale University School of Medicine Department of Psychiatry. He was board president of a child guidance clinic and chairman of a Program Review Committee for the state Department of Mental Retardation. Dr. Makover served as chairman of a hospital psychiatry department, chief of a neuropsychiatry service, and clinical director of psychiatry at a large health maintenance organization. He worked as a consultant in geriatric psychiatry and at a sleep medicine center. He lives in Connecticut with his wife, Janet.

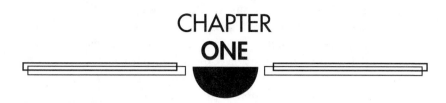

CHAPTER ONE

What Is This Book About?

> For the art is long and life is short
> opportunity fleeting
> experiment dangerous
> judgment difficult.
>
> *Hippocrates*

> If the world were perfect,
> it wouldn't be.
>
> *Yogi Berra*

Introduction

Before computers, before airplanes, before gunpowder, before agriculture, in the unrecorded past of many thousands of years ago, small groups of *Homo sapiens* formed into tribes. They were people like us, with large frontal lobes that allowed them to evaluate, respond to, and modify social behavior and to organize themselves into stratified, hierarchical groups.

Our tribal behavior still persists and pervades every culture, even those aspects we might wish we had left behind. Like those ancient tribes, we even now

- Selfishly compete for property and prestige (social conflict).
- Regard anyone not a member of our "tribe" with suspicion, loathing, and fear (xenophobia).
- Kill each other over territory (genocide).

Our genetic makeup, with all its primitive traits and proclivities, has not evolved throughout those many millennia. Despite our technology

1

and our attempts at civil harmony, we remain subject to the same passions and respond to the same stimuli as our prehistoric ancestors. This roster of unevolved traits also includes our responses to psychological factors, both cognitive and emotional, that create both our mental health and our mental illness and that make us susceptible to psychological stress and to the forces generated in psychological healing.

Those primitive tribal members must surely have vied for status, engaged in intrigue, practiced deception, warred on their neighbors, formed alliances, and exhibited the same variety of individual quirks, habits, and traits that we see today in our contemporaries and in ourselves. Throughout the sweep of history, in large social groups and small families, in casual encounters and stable pairs, whether closely bonded or loosely connected, men and women have always attempted to influence how others thought, felt, and acted. Much of this effort has involved the mandate of social groups to strengthen conformity among their members. Much of it has also taken place in the context of organized religion, and the same struggle to influence behavior animated those who sought political power or commercial success.

Among those early tribal groups, some individuals were recognized as designated experts in behavioral change, with enhanced status and influence as a result of their social position. We can make an educated guess that at least some of these special individuals exerted their powers to minister to the ills of the sick and the dysfunctional. These shamans were designated healers who called on supernatural forces and employed magic rituals to magnify their efforts. If the history of these healers traces back to early primitive tribes, then their work places them among the oldest professions. As shown in Figure 1–1, however, the healer's position in the tribe was both communal and separate. She or he had power just below that of the leader, but the tribe viewed the healer with both fear and respect and sometimes with awe. That ambivalence gave the healer a high status, but at the same time it kept her or him apart from the community, as it does to some extent in our contemporary society.

Over the last century or so, socially approved healers have offered their expertise in behavioral change under the heading of psychological treatment. As successors to those ancient tribal practitioners, we modern healers promise help to those who want to change behaviors identified as personally distressful or socially disruptive. At the beginning of this era of personal assistance, the bulk of these services were consumed by two socioeconomic groups:

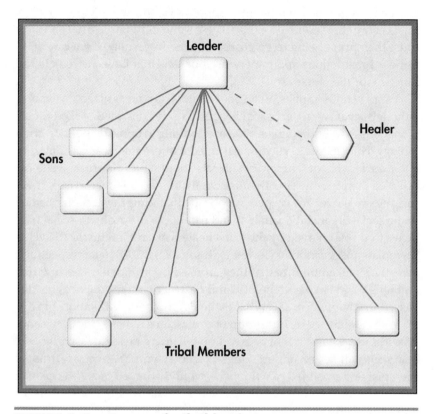

FIGURE 1-1. **Status of tribal healer.**

- The poor and disadvantaged, who often received this "help" involuntarily, and
- The wealthy and privileged, who consumed them as a luxury.

Since the end of World War II, however, more and more people of the middle classes and of ordinary means have accepted this type of healing and have taken advantage of the increasing availability of mental health services.

To meet this rising demand, a separate category of professional healer has emerged: the psychotherapist. Distinct from purveyors of religion and practitioners of medicine, the members of this group come from a number of service professions: medicine, nursing, psychology, social work, physician assistants, and a variety of counseling occupations. Mostly, we are certified and licensed, a postgraduate process that solidifies our social and professional status. Most of our services are compensated (and therefore regulated) through commercial and governmental "third-party" payment programs. Their financial support has encouraged the growth of this sector of the service economy. These same third parties, however, because their primary interest is cost containment and not patient care, have imposed restrictions and paperwork burdens that have altered clinical practice for the worse.

We psychotherapists, like tribal healers, are recognized as experts, although what we are expert in is often loosely construed. Asked for explanations, psychotherapists have been willing to opine on politics, criminology, child-rearing, consumerism, education, the financial markets, and a variety of contemporary subjects about which, in truth, we know no more than anyone else. Because we are offered this special expert status, and are willing to accept it, we occupy that same mysterious position in the social organization, half in and half out of the ordinary social hierarchy, that was enjoyed by the tribal healers of early prehistory. Psychotherapists are even today viewed with some mixture of fear, respect, and awe, the same ambiguity that they aroused in primitive tribes, and that ambiguity can have both helpful and destructive consequences (as discussed in Chapter Three, "What Is the Psychotherapy Relationship?").

Well established as our group of professions may be, the service we provide, *psychotherapy*, is a poorly defined, many-headed, disorganized, and sectarian set of undertakings. Whether you are a newly trained therapist or a seasoned practitioner, you find yourself in a vast ocean of

- Contradictory ideas.
- Controversial claims.
- Conflicting theories.
- Confusing practices.

Surrounding this ocean are mountains of psychotherapy research that present a difficult intellectual task, as published material appears to continually challenge some ideas, support others, and offer up new theories. Faced with this unsettled panorama of competing ideologies, you are naturally inclined to look for a safe harbor in a congenial methodology. Career management is simpler if you select only one modality and concentrate your energies on its theory and practice. Soon, your dedication and your investment of time and resources might incline you not only to ignore other promising ideas but also to defend your chosen path with dogmatic intensity.

At the center of this roiling ocean, however, is an island of common principles and practices that provide a foundation on which all the separate ideologies and methodologies can rest (Figure 1–2). This book is fo-

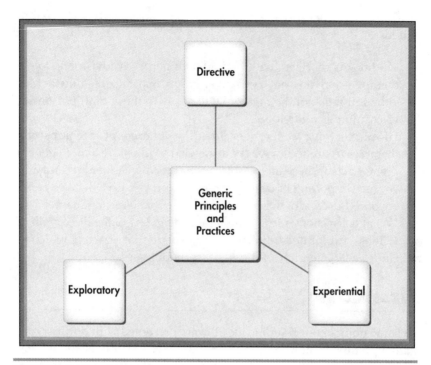

FIGURE 1–2. Generic core.

cused on that central core. Its goal is to identify and explain some of the common ideas and basic concepts that apply to psychotherapy practice in general. This core includes

- A common therapeutic dynamism shared by all psychotherapies.
- A generic psychotherapy, a sort of foundational system from which all other types of psychotherapy develop.
- Techniques that are useful in every methodology.

Familiarity with these core concepts can help you understand

- How the psychotherapy relationship provides the foundation for every methodology.
- The role of the therapeutic alliance in the healing process.
- The central principles all therapies have in common.
- How to organize and carry out treatment to maximize its chances for success.
- How to deal with the common problems any therapy will encounter.

To keep this book to a manageable length, I have imposed two limitations:

- The book is confined to individual treatment—dyadic or one-to-one therapy—and does not try to cover group, marital, or family therapy, although much of the material will apply to those multiperson services, mutatis mutandis.
- I do not survey, examine, or evaluate the hundreds of specific psychotherapies in use today, except as needed to illustrate a more general point. Each of these methodologies has its own adherents and a literature supporting its claims. Tempting as it is, such a detailed task is beyond the scope of this undertaking. Nevertheless, in Chapter Two, "What Is Psychotherapy," I attempt an overview of the three main divisions—exploratory, directive, and experiential—each of which includes a large variety of different methodologies.

First Case

At some point in our training, we all were presented with our first case. Although preparation for this event may have included some reading and (maybe) some direct instruction, for most of us this experience was like learning to swim by jumping into the deep end of the pool.

NORMAN NEOPHYTE

As an example of perhaps a too common experience, we can look over the shoulder of a new psychotherapist—call him Norman Neophyte— as he is about to meet Lisa, his first psychotherapy patient. Lisa is a young woman who was initially evaluated in the outpatient screening clinic of the local hospital with a complaint of "bad nerves." Somehow, her complaint got her seen first by a neurologist, with a negative work-up, before she was referred to the behavioral health service. After three "evaluation" visits at the mental health clinic, she was accepted for psychotherapy and placed on a waiting list. Five weeks later the clinic contacted her and set up her initial appointment. In total, then, nearly three months have elapsed from the time she first applied for help to this first session.

What should we expect after this long delay?

- Lisa must be highly motivated and perhaps in a great deal of emotional distress to accept this bureaucratic postponement. Or maybe she has had to accept the delay because she cannot afford a private referral.

- Lisa came with a (misunderstood) neurological complaint but appears to have readily accepted a mental health referral. Or maybe she is simply following the recommendation of the "experts" in their white coats.
- Lisa's problem may have changed over the several weeks she has waited for help. Or she might even have recovered to some extent, since many people do improve simply by the anticipation of treatment implied by the waiting-list assignment. Sometimes the enforced delay allows the precipitating stress to dissipate, reducing the symptoms that impelled the initial request for help.
- Lisa's estimate of the importance of this meeting and of the professional judgment of the clinical team may have been heightened by the ordeal of several evaluations. Or perhaps she is understandably frustrated and discouraged by the long delay.

All of these factors must have raised her expectations of this final phase of the long process. With the cumulative effects of a neurological consultation, a mental health evaluation, the validation of acceptance for treatment, and the growing anticipation as she awaited her assigned appointment, Lisa might reasonably expect great results.

In honor of the occasion, Norman has worn a tie. He buttons the collar of his blue-and-red checked dress shirt and snugs up the knot of the skinny black knit tie. Before he goes out to the waiting room to greet his new patient, he pauses to review the referral. On his tablet, he logs in, brings up the patient record, and reads the evaluation summary (Figure 1–3).

Norman is assigned to one of the offices in the mental health clinic. The room is about 10 feet by 8 feet, with a desk, a lamp, and two chairs, and is illuminated by overhead fluorescent strip lights (Figure 1–4). On the wall hangs a dusty print of Vincent van Gogh's *Sunflowers*. The window is shielded by a Venetian blind, slats closed. The walls are painted a light institutional green. Norman places his backpack and tablet on the desk and swings the desk chair to face what has to be the patient's chair next to the desk.

Norman and Lisa: First Session

At Norman's invitation, Lisa comes into the room and takes the chair next to the desk. She looks at him expectantly. At this point Norman is thinking

- I don't like this dreary room. She's practically sitting in my lap.
- What's the first thing I should say?

University   Hospital

Mental Health Clinic
Intake Service

Lisa XXXXXXXX
Age: 19
Marital Status: married
Employment: homemaker
Insurance: Blue Cross (husband)
January 6, 2017

EVALUATION SUMMARY

Lisa is a 19-year-old white female, married six months, who presents with a chief complaint

of "nerves." Her husband is a mechanic at an automobile dealership. She is a homemaker. They

married one week after their high school graduation. Alone at home she experiences nearly

constant low-level anxiety punctuated by two or three panic attacks per day. She controls these

by rebreathing into a paper bag. Her anxiety subsides when her husband is home. Her sleep and

appetite are normal, and she is otherwise in good health. A neurology consultation found no CNS

abnormalities. Mental status examination shows an alert, friendly, but restless young woman with

mildly pressured but goal-directed speech. She is well groomed, with somewhat heavy make-up,

dressed in a patterned blouse and dark slacks. Memory is intact. Judgment is age-appropriate.

Estimated IQ is 110–120. She denies depressed mood and suicidal ideation. There is no evidence

of impaired reality testing, hallucinations, or delusions.

Diagnostic impression: Generalized anxiety disorder (300.02)

Plan: Individual psychotherapy

Disposition: waiting list until slot available

FIGURE 1–3.   Evaluation summary: Lisa.

- Am I really expected to "talk" this woman into mental health?
- What should I do and how should I do it?

What can we make of these thoughts?

- First, notice the way the room makes Norman uncomfortable. Chances are Lisa feels the same way. The physical setting is a silent but important factor that can promote or retard the healing process (Chapter Three).

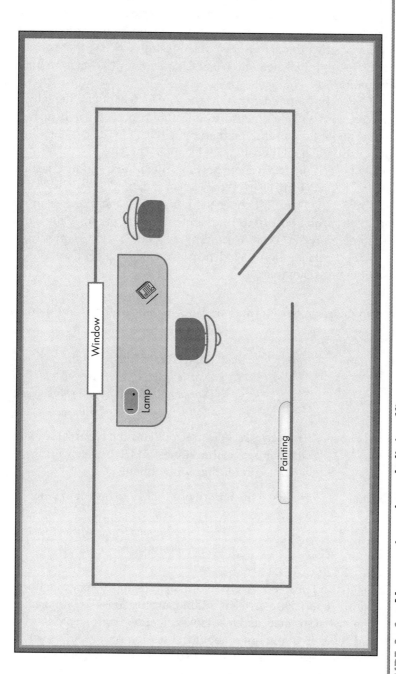

FIGURE 1-4. Norman's assigned clinic office.

- Second, Norman is not prepared with his opening remark, although it may be one of the most important things he says in this first session. How he begins is part of the impression he needs to make to have a positive impact on their relationship and one that starts to structure this initial evaluation (see Chapter Four, "What Is an Initial Evaluation?").
- Next, he lacks confidence that the therapy he will offer will really be effective. Lisa will likely sense his uncertainty and will, in turn, have doubts about how useful the therapy will be. (For discussion of the therapist-patient relationship, see Chapter Three.)
- Finally, he feels uncertain about how to structure and conduct the therapy. In Chapters Four, Five ("What Is a Formulation?"), and Six ("What Is a Treatment Plan?"), I cover the initial assessment, the resulting formulation, and how to use a treatment plan to organize the work. In Chapter Seven ("What Is Communication?") and Chapter Eight ("What Is Collaboration?"), I identify some of the general techniques useful in most therapies.

Meanwhile, we left Norman and his patient in their first therapy minute.

Norman   (*clearing his throat*) So, tell me about yourself.
                        Not a good start. Better would be if
                        Norman made more of an effort to con-
                        nect with Lisa and offer his help.

Lisa   (*looks taken aback*) Don't you have the report? I saw that other person three times, and I've been waiting over a month for this appointment!

Norman   Yes. I have the report, but I'd like to hear it in your own words.
                        Uh-oh, Norman thinks. My first sentence
                        and I'm already having a problem.

Lisa sighs and proceeds to give Norman the same history that he has in the referral report. He asks a few additional questions. The atmosphere is now somewhat strained, and Lisa looks unhappy. Norman picks up his tablet and types in a few notes about the session so far, but mostly to give himself time to think about what to do next. It is not a good idea for Norman to make notes during the session, creating more distance from his patient.

Norman decides to do a mental status examination and asks Lisa the date, then plows through the other standard questions. She appears to have no problems with memory, orientation, cognition, and the rest. The intake evaluation assigned a diagnosis of generalized anxiety disorder even though Lisa also has had panic attacks. On the basis of his evaluation so far, Norman doesn't disagree. He's not sure about what kind of therapy he needs to do, but he decides that medication for the anxiety would be helpful.

Norman	I'd like you to try some medication. It would help you not to feel so nervous.
	This "bottom up" approach and the problems it creates are discussed in Chapter Six.
Lisa	I don't like the idea of taking drugs. I thought *you* were supposed to help me with my nerves.
Norman	Of course. We'll be working on that. But this medication just might make things easier for you.
Lisa	No, I don't want that.
	At least Lisa is forthright in her rejection of this idea. Other patients might passively accept a prescription but never fill it.
Norman	OK, then. Well, I'll see you next week.
	Norman concludes this first meeting without having made progress, but he hopes he can do better next time.
Lisa	I'll have to call back when I know my schedule better.
	Since Lisa is a homemaker with no children to care for, Norman wonders, how busy a schedule could she have? He doubts he will see her again. He feels discouraged.

Norman's first foray into psychotherapy has not gone well, and his patient may not return. Even if she does, Norman does not yet have a clear idea (or, really, any idea) about what he should do for her. His initial evaluation has been unfocused and has not produced much useful information. He has not constructed a single hypothesis from the history he received from the assessment clinic or the information he gathered in the interview. Much of the problem lies in his handling of this first meeting:

- In this barren institutional setting, Norman has not established his professional bona fides. Although he has worn a tie, little in his self-presentation says *I am a professional, and I can do the job.*
- He seats himself and the patient at a desk, which creates an uninviting, authoritarian relationship.
- He begins with an open-ended request for history he already has and that the patient assumes he has. That not only annoys her, it wastes valuable evaluation time.
- He conscientiously performs an unnecessary mental status examination.
- He offers the patient medication without

  1. Completing his assessment (Chapter Four).
  2. Formulating the case (Chapter Five).
  3. Drafting a treatment plan (Chapter Six).
  4. Reaching an agreement with her on how they will work on her problems (Chapter Six).

  No wonder Lisa is reluctant to schedule another session!

Norman and Lisa: Second Session

Nevertheless, to Norman's relief, Lisa makes a second appointment. This time she wears a low-cut blouse and a short skirt. Heavy make-up accentuates her eyes and mouth. Her outfit makes him uncomfortable. He tries not to notice her cleavage.

Norman	I'm glad you came back. How has the week gone for you?
	Norman invites her to provide a chronicle of the interval between sessions, a precedent that might prove problematic in future sessions. Because he has no treatment plan, he has nothing else to focus on.
Lisa	OK, I guess. I'm still having nerves. (*She pauses*) Let me ask you something. Do you like me?
	Lisa voices her concern. Many patients would not raise it so directly, and it would remain unaddressed and corrosive.

Norman   You seem like a nice person. Why do you ask?

> *The right question, because an early problem with the relationship must be dealt with promptly.*

Lisa   You act so distant. I don't know what to tell you or what you want to hear. It's like you don't think I'm interesting.

> *Lisa knows something is wrong but places the blame on herself, perhaps a worthwhile idea for Norman to explore.*

Norman   I do want to help. Right now, I'd like to find out more about you.

> *Instead of trying to explore Lisa's question further, Norman simply answers it, a missed opportunity.*

Norman is again ill at ease as the session begins, in part because his young female patient seems to want to attract his attention to her body, perhaps (as her first question suggests) because she wants him to like her. He is also uncomfortable, however, because he still has no clear idea of how to proceed. He might have recognized that Lisa wants to overcome his perceived coolness with what she hopes is a more attractive physical self-display. Her provocative behavior could give Norman some new and important information about her interpersonal strategies. One hypothesis might be that she feels she cannot interest him as a patient but only as a sexual object. If confirmed, this hypothesis could provide a valuable avenue of inquiry. Norman is too preoccupied with not staring, however, to think about the meaning of her behavior. In Chapter Seven ("What Is Communication?"), I will discuss how to deal with this kind of patient presentation.

Lisa's complaint has zeroed in on the psychotherapy relationship. What type of relationship is it? How does it affect the therapy process? So far, the three parts of the relationship—the therapeutic alliance, the real relationship, and the operational plan, or rather, its absence—as represented in Figure 1–5, add up to only a weak bond with her.

In Chapter Three, I discuss this issue in more detail, examining the therapeutic alliance and the real relationship and how those connections between the two participants contribute to the overall outcome of treatment. What does the patient need to bring to the endeavor? What qualities make a therapist successful? Are therapists born that way, or

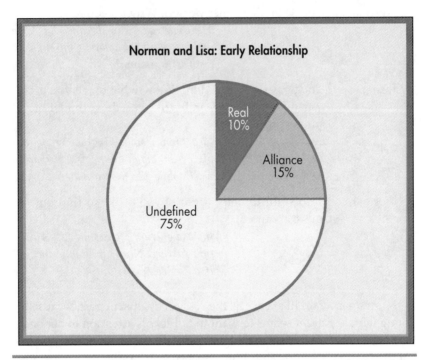

FIGURE 1-5. **Norman and Lisa: psychotherapy relationship.**

can they learn how to be effective and successful? Norman has not been very successful so far. Figure 1–6 represents their connection. As the diagram shows, they each have ideas about the therapy, but most of what they think is as yet unstated, and they do not agree on what it should do or how to accomplish it. Their mutual understanding (area C) is limited and will not support a treatment plan.

In this second session, Norman has reassured Lisa that he is interested in helping her with her problem. He decides to do a more thorough evaluation. Lisa looks pained at this idea, but after Norman expresses an interest in her, she seems willing to go along with what he wants.

Norman now learns that Lisa was an anxious child who had a mild case of school phobia[1]: she would cling to her mother when it was time to go to school, and sometimes she would pretend to be sick so she could stay home. She got over this problem after a few months, but she never liked school. When she entered high school, she began an intense relationship with Gary, the boy who is now her husband. He sounds like a

[1]Also called "school refusal" or, in DSM-5, separation anxiety disorder.

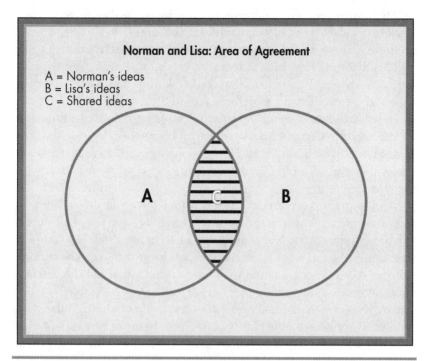

FIGURE 1-6. Norman and Lisa: area of agreement.

hard worker, and he wants her to stay at home while his job supports them. She is bored at home by herself, but her friends from high school are busy with work or college themselves and are not available in the daytime. Gary thinks they should start a family, but she does not feel ready. One reason she has come to the clinic is to delay a decision about getting pregnant until she has recovered from her "nerves" problem.

With this additional history, Norman now has a better picture of Lisa's situation. Unfortunately, he has used two sessions to accumulate what he should have had after one, a waste of valuable time. He wonders whether he should gather more historical information. How much does he need and what will it be used for? In Chapter Four, I examine the assessment: what kinds of information are needed for the psychotherapy to follow? Norman has pursued the standard format of taking a history, but one without any organizing purpose. The narrative is a mere chronology and lacks a connection with Lisa's current symptoms. With more experience, perhaps Norman will begin to construct hypotheses as he hears the history, tentative connections, and explanations that he might use to direct his questions into areas of particular importance.

The second session is at an end, and Lisa indicates she will return next week. After she leaves, Norman writes up his notes. (In Chapter Three, I examine what to record for the legal record and what to leave out.) He decides that next time he will focus on Lisa's loneliness. And her marriage has some early problems that could use attention. Norman is picking out these problem areas without regard to an overall treatment plan and is using the "bottom up" approach. The shortcomings of this method are discussed in Chapter Six. Are these problems the most important aspect of Lisa's overall condition? How do loneliness and marital stress connect with her anxious mood and panic episodes? What result of their work together will represent the optimal outcome of the therapy?

At this point Norman does not consider these questions, but if he did, he would not know the answers. He can only hope they will emerge in later sessions. What Norman should be thinking about is a complete formulation. So far, what he might offer as a formulation can be summarized as: "19-year-old woman with anxiety and early history of school phobia whose recent marriage has left her feeling lonely" (Table 1–1). This statement is only a summary and does not explain why Lisa has these problems, nor does it give Norman any basis to make a treatment plan. In Chapter Five, I review the importance of the formulation and how to make it more than just a summary of the case.

Norman and Lisa: Third Session

Lisa returns for her third appointment. She appears restless and somewhat distracted.

Norman	I'd like to suggest we talk about those lonely feelings you mentioned last time.
	Norman makes a worthwhile attempt at continuity, but he has no defined goal that this subject would fit.
Lisa	(*shrugs*) What's to discuss? I'm lonely because I'm alone all day.
	Lacking an agreement on what they wish to accomplish, Lisa rejects the topic.
Norman	You told me Gary wants you to stay home. Does that mean things aren't going well between you?
	Norman tries again to pick up on information from the previous session, but, again, the question is not part of a treatment plan.

TABLE 1–1. Norman's formulation

Component	Description
Brief summary	19-year-old recently married woman with anxiety
Identified problems	Anxiety (possible panic), boredom, loneliness
Cause-and-effect hypothesis	None
Overall conclusion	None

Lisa	(*looks and sounds angry*) No, everything's fine with us.
	Lisa rejects the second topic too, this time with apparent heat.
Norman	OK then. Why don't you talk about whatever's on your mind.
	Norman is startled by the angry outburst, but he fails to explore it and changes the subject. Once again, the session is not going well. Norman feels somewhat desperate and throws the problem about what to do back onto Lisa.
Lisa	(*still looks angry*) Do you really know what you're doing? We're not getting anywhere.
Norman	I'm trying to help!
	Norman's defensive answer does not address the patient's anger. A better response would be, "You sound angry," a metastatement that could open up a more productive discussion. (For discussion of metacommunication and other generic techniques, see Chapters Seven and Eight.) Searching his memory, Norman comes up with another idea.

Norman   All right. I think this will be helpful: let me tell you
            about some breathing and relaxation exercises you
            can use to control your anxiety problem.

> *Norman wants to do something specific
> to show that he is up to this task. He
> chooses a technical intervention and
> hopes his idea will convince Lisa he does
> know what he's doing. This premature
> intervention may or may not help her
> control her anxiety, but because it is not
> part of an overall plan of treatment, it is
> at best only a symptomatic treatment,
> and at worst it will not help Lisa solve
> the problems that produced her anxiety.*

In this third session Norman has tried to find short-term solutions to
poorly defined problems. The resulting therapy effort is likely to be hap-
hazard and unhelpful. The early meeting between therapist and patient
should be marked by the effects of nonspecific factors that create a feeling of hope and an expectation of benefit (see Chapter Three). After three
sessions Lisa has shown little change and is becoming disillusioned. The
most likely outcome now is that Lisa will drop out of treatment, and who
could blame her?

Compare the two graphs in Figure 1–7. In a successful therapy, hope
and expectations in the first session are high (9 out of 10). Even though
they decrease a bit (7 out of 10) in the next two sessions, they still remain
fairly high. The strength of these feelings predicts a successful outcome.
Indeed, for some patients they may account for the bulk of the success.
With Norman and Lisa, however, Lisa's feelings are quickly diminished
(only 5) by the way Norman handles the initial encounter, and they only
drift lower (to 3 and then 2) over the next two sessions. This pattern suggests that the treatment will not be very successful.

Norman's effort in his third session falls back on technique; specifically, a behavioral intervention. It might help Lisa to control her anxiety
symptoms, but at this point it is not part of an overall plan to help her,
and therefore, Norman's idea does not rest on a good foundation. See
Chapter Six for a review of the steps needed to put together a complete,
useful treatment plan that includes

- The therapy outcome.
- The goals that will lead to it.

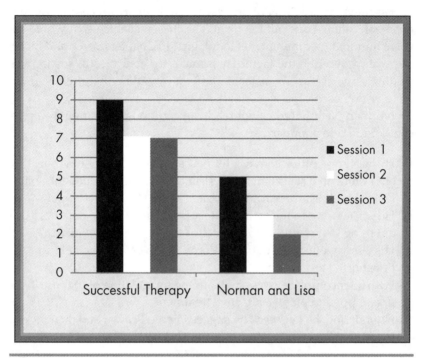

FIGURE 1–7. Norman and Lisa: hopeful expectations.

- The psychotherapy methods likely to help reach those goals.
- The particular techniques needed to implement the therapy process.

In this third session, Norman has once again started an intervention without completing a plan, the unfortunate "bottom up" approach. Table 1–2 shows that Norman's plan is missing most of what is needed.

TABLE 1–2. Norman and Lisa: treatment plan

Component	Description
Final outcome	Undefined
Therapy goals	None set
Methodology	Behavioral treatment
Technique	Relaxation training

Psychotherapies differ in their technical diversity, and as mentioned, this book cannot cover all the many varieties available—that would involve hundreds of different methodologies. In Chapters Seven and Eight, however, I describe the factors that make for a successful session, including some useful *general* techniques that should be helpful whatever therapy is chosen.

Norman Neophyte has not made a propitious beginning as a psychotherapist. To summarize:

- His assigned office conveys little to suggest a professional healing environment: It seats him at a desk and too close to his patient, an unhelpful authoritarian arrangement.
- He wastes time on reviewing history he already has but does not learn anything that would help him better understand his patient.
- His clumsy efforts to initiate therapy fail to establish a helpful relationship.
- With an incomplete assessment and no formulation of the case, he is ill equipped to plan an effective treatment.
- Floundering, he falls back on suggesting medication and then picks a technique, almost at random, that merely hopes to address a symptom.

Altogether, Norman Neophyte has gotten off to a poor start with his first case.

SALLY SKILLFUL

What if Lisa had been assigned to a more experienced therapist? We can call her Sally Skillful. She reads the same evaluation summary (Figure 1–3).

"Uh-oh," she thinks. "A teenage marriage. They usually don't do well."

Sally has not even met her patient, but she has already formed a hypothesis: that an early marriage between two people still in the process of consolidating their own identities and separating from their parents is likely to be fraught with difficulties. This idea may not be important to the case, or it may need revision as more becomes known, but simply having an idea is an advantage. It gives Sally a starting point and an area of concentration around which to organize her initial assessment. The idea could also, of course, be a disadvantage if she allows it to narrow her focus so that she misses or misconstrues important but conflicting information. To formulate a case, you must make, test, revise, discard, and replace hypotheses (see Chapter Five). On balance, Sally's idea is helpful: it places her at the beginning of an important and necessary process that will hopefully lead to a workable treatment plan.

Sally checks out the office before she greets her patient. She rearranges the sparse furniture: she pushes the desk into the corner and moves her chair to the right and the patient chair across the space to the left so that they face each other across the diagonal of the small room (Figure 1–8).

Sally turns off the overhead fluorescent light, brings the lamp to the other side of the desk, and opens the blind to let in some daylight. She puts her bag next to her chair, to mark it as where she sits, but leaves the desk bare. Although she usually does not wear it, she slips into her starched short white coat with her name badge and the clinic logo. Limited as she is by the clinic's physical setup, Sally tries to improve it as much as she can. These nonspecific adjustments are designed to enhance the therapeutic alliance (see Chapter Three):

- She moves the chairs to avoid sitting behind an "authoritarian" desk.
- She designates one of the chairs as "hers."
- She eliminates the "institutional" fluorescent lighting in favor of more natural illumination.
- She dons a coat and badge that will emphasize her professional status.

Sally and Lisa: Initial Interview

Now Sally is ready. In the waiting room she greets Lisa.

Sally	Hi, I'm Sally Skillful. Please come in.
	She could have said, "Hi, I'm Sally," or "Hi, I'm Dr. Skillful (or Ms. Skillful). The first is too informal and the second might be too formal for a young woman just out of high school. Lisa enters the office, and Sally follows.
Sally	(*after they are seated*) I see you had an evaluation last month. Is there anything new since then?
	Sally acknowledges that she has some prior history and does not waste time getting Lisa to recite it again, although she knows she will need more information later in the session.
Lisa	(*smiles*) I'm still the same. I still have my nerves but not as bad. I'm actually feeling a little better.

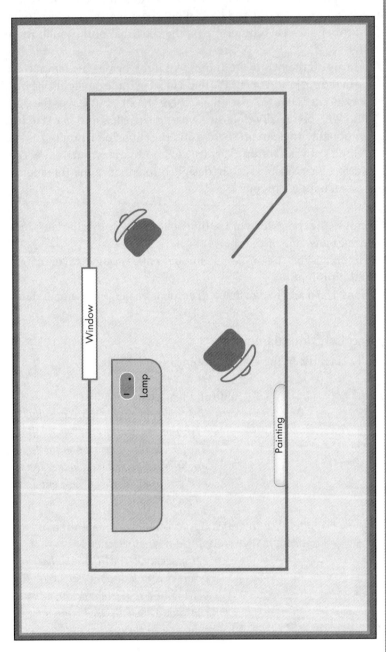

FIGURE 1–8. **Sally's modified clinic office.**

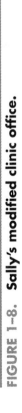

Sally	Good to hear. How about the panic attacks?
	Sally wants to know if the diagnosis of generalized anxiety disorcer is adequate, or if panic disorder might be more accurate.
Lisa	(*thinks a moment*) I had one right after they referred me, but nothing since then. Do you think I'm getting over this problem?
Sally	Sounds like it. People tend to feel better on the waiting list, even though therapy hasn't started. Maybe it's just knowing you're going to get some help.
	Sally acknowledges her improvement and draws attention to the therapeutic alliance.
Lisa	(*leans forward*) What kind of help?
Sally	Let's talk about that. How long have you had problems with your nerves?
	Sally ducks the question of what treatment she intends to recommend because she does not yet know what it should be.

Lisa tells her about her separation anxiety in childhood and the way it came back after she and Gary settled into their new apartment. Sally also learns that she came to the clinic because Gary was pressuring her about getting pregnant, that they had a big fight over it, and that she made an appointment the next day. Sally has identified the event that precipitated the referral, and she notes that it was marital stress, not a panic attack. Now she wants to figure out what she and Lisa should do about it.

Sally	So it's not only the nerves, but also how to deal with Gary?
	Sally tests the hypothesis that Lisa's anxiety is related to problems in the marriage.
Lisa	I guess so. I hadn't really thought about that part before.

Sally   Our time is up. We have to stop, but let's talk next
               time about how we're going to work on these
               problems.

                              Sally introduces a two-sentence formula
                              (Our time is up. We have to stop) that
                              will be helpful when she has to termi-
                              nate future sessions. She also opens the
                              topic of a treatment contract.

Lisa   OK. When can I come back?

In contrast to Norman's initial interview, Sally has made progress:

- She acknowledged the prior evaluation and used the information as a foundation for her assessment.
- She acquired more useful information without going over ground already covered.
- She identified the problem areas and proposed to work out a plan to deal with them.

After Lisa leaves, Sally thinks about a formulation. She knows that the better it is, the more effective will be her treatment plan. Her information at this early stage is limited, and she may have to modify her plan as she learns more about her patient, but she can still generate some working hypotheses.

It seems to Sally that Lisa has a problem with overdependency. She had trouble separating from home to go to school, she married immediately after high school graduation (as if she could not face a future on her own), and she has difficulty being home alone (even though she has made no effort to go out into a more social environment). These ideas constitute a tentative but useful formulation (Table 1–3).

Sally now has a basis on which to construct a treatment plan for Lisa (Table 1–4). The outcome of their work together should be to help her move forward toward adult status. In short, the outcome should be "develop more independence." Sally's initial therapy goals—subject to change—include the following:

1. Achieve more adult independence from her family of origin by completing the normal separation required when an individual establishes a family of procreation.
2. Develop a more independent role in the marriage.

TABLE 1–3. Sally's formulation

Component	Description
Brief summary	19-year-old recently married woman with anxiety
Identified problems	Anxiety (possible panic), pressure by husband to begin family
Cause-and-effect hypothesis	Unresolved dependency fuels fears of separation, isolation
Overall conclusion	Forward progress toward adult independence will help resolve anxiety and marital pressures

TABLE 1–4. Sally and Lisa: treatment plan

Component	Description
Final outcome	Develop independence
Therapy goals	1. Separation from family 2. Marital independence
Methodology	Psychodynamic psychotherapy
Techniques	To be determined

Other possible goals might include readiness for pregnancy and parenthood and consideration of work outside the home, but these objectives are not yet justified by the available history and may not be necessary for a successful course of psychotherapy initiated by a complaint of "nerves." Note that "eliminate anxiety" is not one of Sally's goals. Her hypothesis is that Lisa's anxiety is a symptom of her identified problems and will subside when those problems have improved.

From what she knows of Lisa and her problems at this point, Sally thinks the best type of therapy might be psychodynamic. Lisa's difficulty with individuation seems to reside in unresolved issues from her childhood that have held her back from the normal progression of adult development. An examination of earlier stages and the family environment would be a reasonable way to approach these issues. Where Norman had no overall idea about a therapy plan, Sally has a good starting point and knows what she needs to cover when she sees Lisa again. Although Sally's plan is not yet complete, unlike Norman, she has been able to begin one. Also in contrast to Norman, who attempted to suggest treatments before deciding what he needed to treat, Sally is working "from the top down." She knows what result she wants the therapy to achieve, a result based on a coherent formulation that attempts to explain the "why" of the case. As a consequence, she is more likely to help Lisa to a successful outcome. What it takes to conduct a successful therapy—how to get from the treatment plan to its completion with a good outcome—is covered in Chapter Six, including the need to monitor progress, revise the plan as needed, and end the treatment at the right point.

Norman is hardly to blame for the poor start to his career as a psychotherapist. After all, it is only his first case, and no one has yet told him what to do. So far, nothing in his studies has covered the practical (or even the theoretical) aspects of generic therapy practice. Even if his program had already started to prepare him, however, he would not have all the tools he needs at this early point in his training. Unlike surgeons, therapists rarely get to stand next to an experienced practitioner and learn through a hands-on apprenticeship. Reading about various therapies, although useful as background, does not provide the same learning potential as seeing an actual patient, but even that experience can have limited value. If no one supervises what Norman is doing, it is all too easy for him to make the same mistakes over and over. He could continue to see patients and not incorporate any new ideas and approaches. He would become a more polished and experienced version of his present self but not a more effective and successful therapist. Some of his patients would get better anyway, through changes in the stress levels in their lives or just the natural tendency to healing. Seeing more patients and not doing anything to improve his understanding and his skills, however, would be a disservice to them and a waste of his career. In Chapter Nine ("What Is an Autodidact?"), I will discuss how a combination of experience and new learning can develop and improve therapy skills.

How Norman and Sally conducted their therapies tells us something important about psychotherapy in general.

- How you relate to the patient can be as important as what you do with the patient.
- Some of the factors that create behavior change are not a part of any particular methodology. Instead, they are healing forces that must be present for any methodology to be effective.
- Therapy that follows a plan, whatever that plan might be, is more effective than an unplanned effort that relies on random chance and the application of a particular technique.

Final Thoughts

What this book is about, then, is how to use the basic principles and practices of psychotherapy to improve your competence with any methodology you choose to employ. It covers the essential steps needed for successful practice:

- Establish a therapeutic alliance.
- Make a useful initial assessment.
- Develop an accurate and complete formulation.
- Construct a workable treatment plan.
- Conduct an effective therapy.
- Improve your knowledge and skills.

Psychotherapy is an art whose roots lie deep in the collective unconscious of our species. Despite its elaboration into the hundreds of separate methodologies in current use, its nucleus rests on a few common principles that unite all the different modalities. Therapeutic change results from the combined effects of generic psychotherapy and a specific strategy—psychodynamic, cognitive, existential, and all the others. This generic psychotherapy is the subject of this treatise, along with a related group of useful phenomena that are central to its daily practice. These core abilities will form a solid foundation for becoming an expert in psychotherapy, and therapists who understand them will be more effective and successful at whatever particular methodologies they choose to employ in their work.

Key Points

- The social role of psychological healer has its roots in early human tribal relationships.
- Certain common principles provide the foundation for all psychotherapies.
- Generic psychotherapy includes the therapeutic environment, the social status of the therapist, and the positive relationship between the therapist and the patient.
- Principles and practices of generic psychotherapy must be learned, along with the strategies and techniques of specific methodologies.

- Initial assessment, formulation, and "top down" treatment plans improve the efficiency and effectiveness of psychotherapy.
- The practice of psychotherapy is an art rather than a science, but a familiarity with its foundational principles will improve every therapist's success.

CHAPTER
TWO

What Is Psychotherapy?

Myself when young did eagerly frequent
Doctor and Saint, and heard great Argument
About it and about: but evermore
Came out by the same door as in I went

Omar Khayyám

I wish I had an answer for that because
I'm really tired of answering that question.

Yogi Berra

Introduction

The answer to the question "What is psychotherapy?" usually includes some reference to "talk" and to "psychology" and perhaps to the idea of "analysis." A dictionary might define it as the use of psychological methods to treat mental and emotional disorders. On the one hand, this simple definition leaves out any consideration of the complex relationship involved or the multitude of therapeutic variations. On the other hand, unnecessary complexity can obscure important aspects of psychotherapy that are simple and straightforward. It may not be possible to construct a definition that covers all of the different methodologies that lay claim to the "psychotherapy" title, but it is worthwhile to define the core qualities, the basic parts of any psychotherapeutic modality. In this chapter, I examine those generic features.

Another definition, although a circular one, is that psychotherapy is whatever a psychotherapist does. That definition begs the question "What is a psychotherapist?" A related question might be "Are psychotherapists professionals?" Although the term *professional* has broadened to include almost any distinct occupation (professional bowler, professional carpenter, professional typist), the designation, in its classical sense, refers to a person who

- Has undergone special training to acquire expertise in a particular field of endeavor.
- Employs predominantly intellectual skills that require the consistent exercise of judgment and discretion.
- Is guided by a set of standards, covering both conduct and ethics, specific to the occupational group.
- Is certified by a recognized authority, often comprising members of the occupational group.
- Is often distinguished by a set of social designators (the physician's white coat, the judge's robes), although these are not limited to or reserved for the group's members.

Given these criteria, we can ask again, is psychotherapy a profession? The traditional specialties—psychiatry, psychology, social work, nursing, physician assistant—clearly fit the definition. On the margins of this core group, however, is a collection of occupations that lack one or more of those professional requirements. Individuals in these occupations may call themselves psychotherapists, or they may designate their work by such titles as pastoral counselor or life coach. *Psychotherapist*, then, is not a distinct profession but rather a collection of professions and semiprofessions. Nevertheless, the generic principles and practices of psychotherapy apply across the spectrum.

Terminology

Given the variety of occupational claims to the title of psychotherapist, it is necessary to define the terms used in this book. In any psychotherapy, a trained mental health professional provides a healing service to a recipient suffering from psychological distress.

- The trained professional could be called the healer, the provider, the psychotherapist, or the analyst, but I will use *therapist*.
- The service is almost always provided in discontinuous allotments of time that could be called meetings, appointments, visits, or encounters, but I will call them *sessions*.
- The recipient of the service might be called a subject, an analysand, a client, a customer, or even (by corporate health care administrators) an "income stream," but I prefer *patient*.

The focus will be on the two-person unit: a dyad. The two meet on a schedule in an appropriate setting for a specified amount of time. Although variations of all three conditions are possible,

- The schedule is usually the therapist's schedule.
- The setting is usually the therapist's office.
- The time allotted is usually one hour and often less.

The psychotherapeutic relationship (discussed in the next chapter) has certain characteristics that set it apart from other dyads, such as those found, for example, in

- Long friendships.
- Sibling pairs.
- Married couples.

but *some* of these characteristics are also found in other two-person relationships, such as

- Coach-athlete.
- Priest-penitent.
- Programmer-user.

In other respects, however, the psychotherapy relationship is unique.

Less often, the psychotherapy unit exceeds two and comprises a therapist and

- a spousal pair (marital therapy);
- a multigenerational kinship (family therapy); or
- an assembly of unrelated individuals (group therapy).

Some of the same conditions and rules may still apply, mutatis mutandis, to these larger groups as well (Table 2–1).

Background

The discovery in 2013 of a cave in South Africa that contained hundreds of carefully arranged skeletons of Middle Paleolithic humans, placed in positions that suggested the outcome of a funeral ritual, was considered evidence that even this most primitive tribe buried its dead. If true, then it is also likely that they practiced psychotherapy.

TABLE 2–1. Psychotherapy relationships

Number of participants	Composition: therapist plus	Type of therapy	Intensity of relationship with therapist
Two	One individual	Dyadic (Individual)	High
Three	Committed pair	Triadic (Couples)	Moderate
Four plus	Two or more generations	Multigenerational (Family)	Low
Four plus	Three or more unrelated individuals	Transactional or interpersonal (Group)	Low

- A culture that has a concept of an afterlife is apt to also have healing rituals, usually expressed in social gatherings and through the use of what we might call "magic."
- The legitimacy and authority for these gatherings would rely on the tribe's mythology, its supernatural beliefs, and their derived customs.
- The healing ritual might employ rhythmic music, dance, or mind-altering drugs to help evoke strong emotions in the sufferer.
- In this special setting, a designated healer—a priest, a shaman, a medicine woman or man—would try to relieve a tribal member of a mental, emotional, or spiritual affliction.
- The healer would assume the clothing and symbols that designated this special status and might engage in a ceremony and perhaps enter an altered mental state (like a trance) in order to access the forces needed to heal the sufferer.

As I noted in the previous chapter, the paleohealer would have been treated with a mixture of reverence, awe, caution, and unease. Those in touch with supernatural forces evoked both respect and anxiety in the group. Today, mental disturbances still create unease in the social group, especially if the sufferer's behavior appears unpredictable. Consequently, those who attempt to help them are also viewed with doubt and suspicion. Tell others your profession and what you do and they might become wary, as if you might uncover their secrets ("Can you read my mind?") or say something disconcerting or impolite.[1] The am-

---

[1]I try to reassure people who react this way by saying, semiseriously, "Don't worry. I only do that stuff when I'm getting paid for it."

bivalence with which society views psychotherapists is also conveyed by our frequent inclusion in jokes, our representation in comedy skits and as evil schemers in films and novels, and in the use of derogatory terms such as "shrink," a shortened version of "headshrinker."

Our modern culture began to acknowledge this process of psychological healing in the late eighteenth century. A German astronomer, Franz Anton Mesmer, believed he could transfer energy between inanimate and animate objects (*animal magnetism*), and he developed a hypnotic procedure (*mesmerism*) to dispel the symptoms of "hysteria." Mesmerism and its practitioners were discredited in 1784 by a prestigious Royal Commission because they could demonstrate no physical basis for what they did.[2] Today, some of that same skepticism remains. While we may not be investigated by a Royal Commission, we are often chided for the lack of hard evidence to support what we do. And even in these enlightened times, some think of us as charlatans or necromancers, or worse.

That old diagnostic category, hysteria, covered a broad array of psychic ills, among them—in today's terminology—fugue states, dissociative identity disorder, somatic symptom disorder, conversion disorder, posttraumatic stress disorder, and borderline personality. Mesmerism was a broad-spectrum treatment. Sigmund Freud tried this new "hypnosis," found its effects did not last, and instead created a method he called *psychoanalysis*. We can already see how this modern approach parallels primitive healing rituals. Psychoanalysis

- Envisions an unknowable powerful force (the unconscious).
- Requires a special place (the analytic office).
- Defines unique roles for the healer and sufferer (as designated by a chair and a couch).
- Evokes strong emotions (the transference).
- Employs a ritual (free association).
- Can be performed only by a designated healer (Freud would only recognize a physician who had undergone analysis himself).
- Requires the healer (the analyst) to enter an altered mental state (free-floating attention).

---

[2]Benjamin Franklin, in France representing the colonies in the War of Independence, was a member of the Commission. It concluded that Mesmer's results were due to "the power of imagination" or what we might call the power of suggestion.

- Promises relief from mental or emotional distress (Freud hoped he could turn neurotic suffering into common misery).
- Aspires to attain spiritual goals (the full realization of the self's potential).

Today, among the diverse cultures of the world, there are *hundreds* of separate psychotherapies. They all share some of these ancient common attributes, and the proponents of each methodology claim (not inaccurately) that it will produce therapeutic results. This multiplicity suggests that there is no one "right answer." Does this mean that the methodologies themselves are merely window dressing, empty procedures without meaning or importance? I prefer to think that this rich diversity suggests that the benefits of each are more selective; that is, each type of therapy might work best within a particular culture, with its distinctive social structure, for a particular patient, with his or her unique set of problems. The parallels between ancient rituals and modern psychotherapy should reassure us that a phenomenon that has sustained human cultures for tens of thousands of years will be a worthwhile endeavor for the modern practitioner, albeit under much different conditions and expectations.

Methodologies

To understand modern psychotherapy, then, we need to look into these phenomena more closely. Suppose you were the psychotherapist in the following encounters:

- Elizabeth, a 30-year-old homemaker, highly anxious, drives across a bridge, jaw clamped and hands white-knuckled on the wheel. In the passenger's seat you remind her to control her breathing and to lean back.
- Matthew, a 24-year-old graduate student, lies on a couch talking discursively about a remembered dream. You sit behind him, out of sight, and listen intently but in silence.
- Gregory, a 75-year-old retired attorney, paces the floor, ruminating about the end of his life. You sit nearby, quiet except for occasional statements that clarify his ideas or acknowledge his feelings.
- Vincent, a 28-year-old former Marine, reimagines the IED attack that killed two of his buddies, destroyed his Humvee, and left him blind in one eye. You guide him through the memory with hypnotic suggestions.

- Julia, a 54-year-old administrative assistant, weeps as she discusses her husband's indifference to her feelings. You intervene to point out a logical inconsistency in her account.

In each of the above examples you have made use of a particular type of psychotherapy:

- For Elizabeth's phobia you employ a behavioral approach.
- You and Matthew are engaged in psychoanalysis.
- To help Gregory you offer an existential ear.
- Hypnosis is one of your techniques to facilitate Vincent's struggle to overcome posttraumatic stress.
- In accordance with cognitive therapy principles, you challenge Julia's negative overgeneralizations.

Assume you have all of those skills. In each case you have elected to use one approach out of many. You had various different psychotherapies to choose from, each with a unique structure—a set of specific ideas and procedures—that distinguishes it from the others. Your choice of which therapy to use relied on your mastery of a select few of these many methodologies and, even more important, on your *expectation* that your work with your patient will have a good outcome.

Common Features

As you might expect, for all of these psychotherapies to be capable of producing a good result, they must share a core set of common features. These common elements have been recognized as the placebo effect, nonspecific factors, and agents of therapeutic change.

PLACEBO EFFECT

The first core feature, the *placebo effect* (sometimes called the *placebo response*), refers to the beneficial results obtained from a treatment known to be inert or inactive, the proverbial "sugar pill." Even though inactive, a placebo can cause real changes in physiology, including alterations in brain waves and body chemistry. Placebos can be used for good purposes or bad.

- A placebo can temporarily reduce or relieve pain without risking side effects or drug dependence.

- A placebo response to a fake cancer drug sold by an unscrupulous "drug company" may relieve subjective symptoms but delay effective treatment.

Placebos seem to work by a self-hypnotic mechanism, sometimes called "the power of suggestion." Some degree of placebo effect is present in a variety of treatments.

- If patients are offered a low-price generic drug and then a higher-priced brand name version, they will show a better response to the more costly drug, even though both versions are pharmacologically identical.
- Larger pills work better than smaller ones, and "hot" colored pills work better than "cool" ones.
- A "sham" treatment—for example, a mammary artery graft for coronary heart disease—can bring about (at least temporary) improvement.[3]
- The authority of the prescriber—the physician in her white coat or the auspices of a prestigious hospital—enhances the treatment response.

In psychotherapy, the placebo effect shows up indirectly, since we do not have diagnostic instruments or laboratory tests to document progress.

- Some patients get better after an evaluation interview followed by placement on a waiting list, even though they have received no formal treatment.
- Patients may show significant relief from symptoms early in the psychotherapy, too soon, presumably, for it to have its intended effect.
- Placebo-accelerated progress throughout a course of treatment may be stimulated by the patient's increased anticipation of benefit.
- Prominent therapists or those who hold a prestigious position can expect better results from the placebo effect. So can regular therapists who are associated with a respected institution or who work in a professionally important building. The therapist who looks "professional" will also boost the placebo effect.

---

[3]Relief from angina (chest pain) was the same in patients who received the graft and those who underwent the sham surgical procedure in which no grafting was performed.

- A new psychotherapy, or one with a status that is enhanced by positive word of mouth or media publicity, will gain in effectiveness from its novelty or heightened prestige due to a placebo response.
- A therapist's good reputation in the community creates a placebo-enhanced impact for his or her patients.
- Therapists who have high confidence in a treatment will have better results from the increased placebo response than from one about which they are uncertain.

Placebo benefits, in psychotherapy as elsewhere, are powered by the expectations of the therapist and the patient, and they can translate into permanent improvements (Table 2–2).

TABLE 2–2. Beneficial effects of placebo

Source	Result	Beneficial factor
Consultation	Complete recovery	"Magical" status
Early therapy	Symptom relief	Enhanced expectations
Professional status, therapist	Strong healing influence	Increased belief
Publicized methodology	Greater rate of improvement	Increased hopefulness

NONSPECIFIC FACTORS

The second core element, *nonspecific factors*, comprises a set of experiences shared both by psychological therapies and by other cultural healing procedures. In 1961, Jerome Frank laid out the necessary conditions needed to recover from psychological impairment. They included a widely variable set of social and cultural activities with common characteristics.[4] The targeted sufferers could be troubled by social isolation, religious despair, physical paralysis, mental disease—indeed, any manner of mental disorder or dysfunction. The healer was a person recognized as an expert with special powers, including social status, religious faith, magical powers, or psychological know-how. The healer's ministra-

---

[4]Frank JD, Frank JB: *Persuasion and Healing: A Comparative Study of Psychotherapy*, Third Edition. Baltimore, MD, Johns Hopkins University Press, 1991.

tions usually included emotional activation, rhetoric, ritual, and other persuasive techniques. These forces were equally at work in

- Every school of psychotherapy.
- Faith healing (religious revivalism and cults).
- Magic rituals that invoked the supernatural and magic.
- Self-help books.
- "Telecommunications" counseling (Frank's book predated computers, mobile devices, and the Internet).

Frank's thesis—that a religious shrine or a tribal ceremony had the same therapeutic status as a psychotherapy office and that an evangelist or a shaman had the same healing influence as a psychoanalyst—originated in his observation that all of these socially accepted forms of psychological healing had features in common. Looking at two-person situations, dyads—like a faith healer and a sufferer, an evangelist and a sinner, a therapist and a patient—he identified four effective characteristics offered in each of these interactions:

1. A *relationship* with a person considered to have the ability to heal. The relationship encourages both emotional expression and open, revealing speech.
2. A special, safe *environment* that verifies the healer's competence and prestige.
3. An *explanation* (or "myth") that makes sense of the emotional distress and confusion ("demoralization," Frank called it) experienced by the sufferer.
4. A *procedure* or system (a "ritual") through which the healer can help the sufferer recover and return to health.

If we apply these findings to psychotherapy, the common, nonspecific factors are

- A competent, recognized therapist whose social standing derives from training, certification, and experience (the healer).
- A patient motivated to receive help for emotional, personal, or social problems (the sufferer).
- A sanctioned association based on voluntary participation and payment for services rendered (the relationship).
- A private, safe, and confidential setting, usually the therapist's office (the environment).

- Their collaborative belief that participation in the therapeutic process will lead to relief from the patient's troublesome problems (the myth).
- A process (or methodology) to be followed in order to achieve the beneficial result (the ritual).

These nonspecific features of a healing paradigm are *necessary* for a successful therapy, but they are usually not *sufficient*. They must be matched with the specifics of a particular methodology. It may be tempting to relegate the specific therapies to the status of mere epiphenomena, interchangeable procedures that are not in themselves effective but that allow the nonspecific forces to work. A coherent methodology, however, is also *necessary* in order to achieve long-term benefits, although it, too, is not *sufficient* alone. One way to think about the way these two therapeutic elements work is that the nonspecific factors are the fuel and the specific methodology is the engine. Without the fuel, the engine is immobile. Without the engine, the fuel is inert. Together, the nonspecific factors and the methodology are necessary *and* sufficient to bring about therapeutic change (Table 2–3).

TABLE 2–3. Nonspecific healing forces in psychotherapy

Nonspecific component	Psychotherapy equivalent
Relationship with designated healer	Therapeutic alliance
Special safe environment	Psychotherapy office
Coherent explanation of suffering (myth)	Psychological theory
Required process of healing (ritual)	Therapeutic methodology

No one knows what proportion of a patient's recovery can be credited to the placebo response and other nonspecific factors and how much improvement depends on the methodology employed. Patients can "recover" after a single session or even while waiting for their first appointment. Estimates of the impact of nonspecific factors range from 40% to 70%, but a reasonable guess is that these factors account for about half. What this estimate means to your work with the average patient is that even with the advantage of these healing forces, you and your patient are only about halfway to achieving a good therapeutic outcome. You will also need to have mastered the appropriate methodology to complete the job (Figure 2–1).

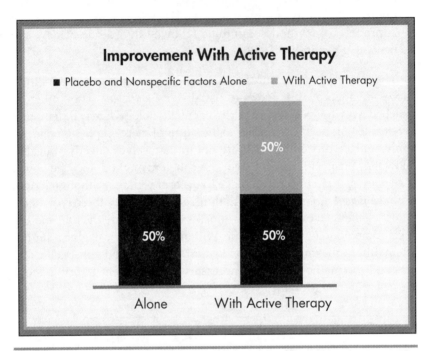

FIGURE 2–1. **Comparison of improvement with nonspecific factors and placebo effect alone and with active therapy.**

Some patients, however, *will* get better solely because of the placebo effects and the nonspecific factors. For them, these forces account for 100% of the result, although these patients are often healthier people with a temporary intercurrent problem, usually stress related. For others, who may be more severely disabled, these factors will contribute less than half to their "healing," but they will often facilitate these patients' cooperative engagement in the treatment that will then account for most of their recovery. Whatever the contribution of these forces to the outcome, whether it is a little or a lot, the rest depends on your experience and skill and on the motivation of your patient. In partnership, they create the maximum opportunity for the patient's improvement.

AGENTS OF THERAPEUTIC CHANGE

In addition to the placebo response and Frank's nonspecific conditions, each methodology, if it is an effective therapy, appears to share certain

TABLE 2–4. General therapeutic factors in psychotherapy

Healing paradigm (Frank)	Placebo response enhancements	Nonspecific factors within therapy (Karasu)
1. A socially respected and approved leader	A socially approved therapist	
2. A safe, special environment	The therapist's high interest and confidence	A strong emotional component
3. A coherent explanation (myth)	The patient's hope and expectation of benefit	A systematic rational explanation
4. A restorative procedure (ritual)	A recognized, well-regarded methodology	A methodology that promotes behavioral change

fundamental underlying requirements (Table 2–4). Karasu identified three "therapeutic change agents"[5]:

1. *Affective experiencing.* The process must elicit the *emotional* content of whatever problems the patient brings to therapy. It may result in sudden, strong surges of affect (catharsis or "abreaction") that by themselves bring only temporary relief, or it may release more sustained but less intense emotions that drive the therapeutic work and enhance the persistence of new behaviors (compare Frank's permissive relationship).
2. *Cognitive mastery.* The methodology must provide an intellectual framework that makes sense of whatever difficulties the patient has had in life and that provides a *rational basis* for their origin (compare Frank's myth). The rational explanation may hypothesize that unresolved childhood conflict creates adult symptoms (psychodynamic) or that automatic thoughts (overlearned self-statements) produce maladaptive behavior (cognitive) or that individual turmoil results from rec-

[5]Karasu TB: "The Specificity Versus Nonspecificity Dilemma: Toward Identifying Therapeutic Change Agents." *American Journal of Psychiatry* 143:687–695, 1986.

ognition of the tragic facts of human life (existential). Based on this explanation, the therapy proposes to ameliorate those difficulties.

3. *Behavioral regulation.* The therapeutic effort must bring about significant and long-lasting change in some or all of the *behaviors* through which the patient's problems are expressed (compare Frank's ritual). Although the mechanisms by which this change is effected differ, the requirement of *positive behavioral change* defines the desired improvement.

Clinical Example

To illustrate this psychotherapeutic change, consider one of the patients, Elizabeth, mentioned earlier in this chapter. You, the therapist, accompany her as she drives fearfully across a bridge. Here is the beginning of your first session with her, two weeks earlier:

You	Good morning. What can I do for you?
Elizabeth	I'm afraid of driving, especially over bridges. I can't drive across the Mianus River Bridge. It's on I-95, near my home. I can't go a lot of places because I can only drive north, away from the bridge. So I want to get over it. My doctor said you were a specialist in phobias.
	The referral identifies you as a socially approved therapist and endows you with a special healing power.
You	I am, but let me find out a little more about your situation. Why that particular bridge?
Elizabeth	Maybe you don't remember, but a section of it collapsed a while back. People died.
You	How far back was that?
Elizabeth	1983.
You	A long time ago! Have you been afraid of it all this time?
Elizabeth	No. It started last year when I saw a news story that said our bridges were being neglected and they were getting more risky all the time. The funny

thing is they fixed that bridge after it fell, and now it's OK. It's probably one of the safest around. But every time I think about crossing it, I get really nervous, and it's getting worse. And now a friend of mine has moved, and the only way I can go to see her is over that one bridge.

> *As you gather additional history, you learn that Elizabeth's mother suffered a postpartum depression after her birth and could not provide adequate nurturance during the first few months of her life. This perinatal deficit has made her a more dependent person, and because the trauma occurred at such an early point in her life, the result may be highly resistant to therapeutic intervention. As an adult, Elizabeth can be whiney, clinging, and lacking in self-confidence. She knows it is a problem, but she does not want help with that ("That's just how I am"). She does acknowledge that since she stopped driving, the dependent behaviors have been worse. You agree to help her with the phobia.*

You   I want you to try something: close your eyes, and in your mind picture driving across the bridge.
> *You initiate a healing ritual.*

Elizabeth   (*with eyes closed*) I'm nervous already!
> *The procedure mobilizes a strong emotion.*

You   On a scale of 1 to 100, where 100 is the worst, how nervous are you?

Elizabeth   85!

You   OK. Let's see if we can bring that down to 25 or less. Between now and when I see you next week, I want you to do this exercise three times a day: Pick a quiet moment when you feel calm to start with and imagine driving across that bridge. Do it for five minutes. Write down the date and time and the number from 1 to 100, so we can review it next time. Can you do that?

You introduce a restorative procedure.

Elizabeth   Are you sure that will help?

You   Your fear of crossing the bridge is something you learned, even though we don't know how that happened. This treatment approach will help you unlearn it, one step at a time. Next week we'll talk about step number two.

You briefly describe the systematic rationale (the myth).

If we had developed a formulation for Elizabeth's problem, we might have considered the following ideas:

- Elizabeth's fear of crossing the bridge has a kernel of truth: sometimes, rarely, bridges do fall, as this one did years earlier, and occasional news reports remind us that deferred maintenance on bridges may create structural failures that make them unsafe. Her fear is highly exaggerated, especially because this bridge has been repaired, but not delusional.
- Perhaps her phobia is Pavlovian: some unrelated anxiety, paired with the unconditioned response of crossing the bridge, set up the phobia as a conditioned response, reinforced by her pattern of avoidance.
- Or a psychodynamic etiology might postulate a symbolic basis for her fear, rooted in some unresolved early trauma. With the behavior therapy used in this case, however, we do not need to know how it came into existence; our treatment method is oriented to present-day relearning.
- Elizabeth adapted to the limitations the phobia imposed until her friend moved to the other side of the bridge. Her dependent character traits may have made her more vulnerable, and the secondary gain (the benefits of being "sick" and needing help) may have contributed. In this behavioral approach, we ignore those antecedents and concentrate only on the immediate problem.

The next week, Elizabeth returns to say she did the exercise, and her score is now 30. She has also, on her own, driven south on the interstate (toward the bridge) but had to get off at the exit before the bridge. When you offer to go with her, she is surprised and worried that she will not make it, but she agrees to do it. With you in the passenger seat, she manages to cross the bridge and has less trouble on the return trip.[6]

Consider the generic elements involved in this treatment process.

- In your "hands-on" session you have directed Elizabeth to enter a phobic situation (crossing the bridge) that arouses anxiety, a strong *emotion*.

- On the basis of your authority, your expert status, she has accepted your idea (the *rationale*) that a controlled, modified exposure will negate the phobia, so her future behavior with regard to crossing bridges will be easier.

- Your presence in the car (a bit of magic *ritual* from your status as a *healer*, because your presence will not prevent a bridge collapse) makes her feel safer. More important: poor nurturance in infancy by a depressed mother may have left her with fears of abandonment. With you beside her, if the car should stall on the bridge, she will not be alone. By temporarily meeting this unexpressed and "unconscious" fear you allow her to face the more immediate and concrete (no pun intended) fear of bridge failure.

Elizabeth is also helped by her trust in you, your interest in her welfare, your professional status, and your implied belief that she is strong enough to undergo this ordeal. The effect of this relationship, the therapeutic alliance, is discussed in the next chapter.

After she has overcome the phobia, Elizabeth becomes less dependent. Her whining and clinging behaviors diminish, and her confidence increases. Experience shows that alleviating one type of problem may benefit another that was not the target of a therapy effort. If her personality disorder was a pot of boiling water, mastering the fear of the bridge lowers the flame so that the water stops boiling and merely simmers. The dependency trait was inborn but magnified by a lack of maternal nurturance. While Elizabeth will not be "cured" of this trait, overcoming the phobia helps improve her older problem. This effect has important implications for treatment planning, as discussed in Chapter Six.

As Karasu's change agents predict, the behavior therapy protocol is successful and changes the previous *behavior* of avoidance into one of

---

[6]As the technology for "virtual reality" becomes available, perhaps Elizabeth would make this trip wearing a headset and you both can enjoy the comfort of your office.

confrontation and mastery. In this behavioral paradigm, the damage done by the lack of nurturance in infancy, which might be of primary importance in a psychodynamic psychotherapy, is irrelevant. Nevertheless, Elizabeth's success in the behavioral exercise promotes a sense of mastery, increases her self-confidence, allows her greater freedom of movement, and improves her self-image. These gains, in turn, make her feel less dependent—a secondary benefit of the treatment. In contrast, a long course of psychodynamic therapy focusing on the origins of her overdependency might result in increased independence but never allow her to overcome her bridge phobia (Table 2–5).

TABLE 2–5. Comparison of therapies for Elizabeth

	Behavior therapy	Psychodynamic therapy
Target problem	Simple phobia	Overdependence
Modality	Directive	Exploratory
Method	In vivo exposure	Interpretive
Result	Phobia overcome Less dependent	Increased independence

A Working Definition

Every year, millions of people seek out and receive psychotherapy, although this large number is only a small fraction of those who could benefit. A majority of patients report that the experience helps them, but what, exactly, is this remarkable experience? It cannot be merely "talk." Frank's thesis gives us general characteristics for all healing states, but we need to define psychotherapy's specific properties. These properties are

- *Transaction.* The process of any therapy requires at least two people who exchange information within a shared relationship and who interact on an interpersonal level. The relationship differs from family or friendship connections because
  - ➤ The patient hires you and pays for the service.
  - ➤ You provide the skills, direction, and overall management of the endeavor.

  The result is a complex contract that combines financial, personal, and social obligations into what becomes a professional collaboration.

- *Change.* A primary tenet of this professional collaboration is your commitment to ameliorate the patient's impaired or dysfunctional psychological condition. A successful outcome of the therapy will mean that the problem behaviors will be modified or eliminated and often will be replaced by behaviors that are more functional and successful.
- *Behavior.* Psychological experiences can take a multitude of forms: traits, emotions, somatizations, dreams, fantasies, memories, perceptions, insights, cognitions, and the like. Therapeutic work may examine and utilize all of these phenomena, but none is an end in itself. The only "currency" in psychotherapy is the patient's behavior; everything else is of use only when it is instrumental to a particular therapeutic modality.
- *Power.* Any interpersonal activity must occur in a power framework. Our societies, our communities, our families are stratified: some individuals have more influence and authority than others. Institutions and places of employment contain similar hierarchies. Dyads rarely reflect an even distribution of power; almost always, one member of the pair predominates over the other. Over time, or with changes in conditions, the balance of power can fluctuate, shift, or even reverse, but at a given moment that balance usually favors one side over the other. In a successful psychotherapy relationship, the balance of power must favor the therapist.

In this definition, then, psychotherapy is a *transactional* method to *change* one or more *behaviors* through an asymmetrical *power* relationship. For Elizabeth, our patient with a phobia, for example, these factors are described in Table 2–6. We can examine each of these components in more detail.

TABLE 2–6. Psychotherapy factors for Elizabeth

Component	Description
Transaction	Patient provides history of avoidance (phobia) Therapist provides explanation ("learned fear")
Change	Approach instead of avoidance
Behavior	Visualize approach Physical approach with support
Power	Persuasion prompts approach in spite of fear

TRANSACTION

- A psychotherapy *transaction* is a communicative exchange. The relationship between the participants may be thought of as a communication conduit, a kind of two-way street. In one direction, from the patient, traffic is heavily weighted toward information and emotion, both historical data and subjective reports. From the other, from your direction, it is primarily investigation, commentary, and instruction.
- The communication usually involves not only conversation, or verbal interaction, but also, and of equal importance, nonverbal exchanges. For example, a nonverbal (and symbolic) exchange is the payment you receive for your services. Most communication is content-based, focused on topics relevant to the patient's treatment plan. Some of the communication conveys relationship meaning; for instance, your unconditional positive regard. Therapeutic communication, then, contains emotional meaning and behavioral significance, as well as social and cultural messages.
- Both participants continually screen and edit their communications:
  - ➢ The patient rarely reveals every thought or feeling on the subject under review.
  - ➢ You restrict your responses and interventions through the exercise of clinical judgment and, in the best case, in accordance with a predetermined treatment plan.
- This communicative exchange is *unbalanced*. It results from an uneven distribution of information.
- The degree of imbalance varies with the type of therapy. The ratio of the patient's production to that of yours is often 2:1 or 3:1 or greater, depending on the kind of therapy in which you are engaged. A behavioral therapy, for example, may require a greater amount of instruction, direction, encouragement, and commentary from you, and your share of the total communication time thus enlarges. In classical psychoanalysis, you, the analyst, may remain silent for days or weeks at a time, and thereby claim only a tiny fraction of the exchange.
- Since each type of therapy has its own characteristic imbalance, a significant change in the degree of imbalance often signals a developing problem with the therapy. For example, the patient in psychoanalysis may go silent, so that neither of you speaks for days. Less dramatic: a patient who has been helpfully vocal about her life may gradually shift to talking about fashion or current events; as personal communication dries up, progress in the therapy slows.

CHANGE

Psychotherapeutic improvement requires behavioral *change*. The behaviors identified as targets of the therapeutic work must be modified for the therapy to be a success. Even a well-motivated patient, however, will find change hard to accomplish. Change is uncomfortable, and the presumably better result of the effort is not certain. Change creates anxiety, even in healthy people.

- The patient's symptomatic behavior represents an accommodation to unhealthy conditions, but although it is an uneasy solution, it is nevertheless one that has worked up to now, at least to some extent. For example, a patient with compulsive rituals may not like the burden of checking the stove and the doors or counting the number of steps, but doing so binds anxiety and trades time spent checking for temporary calm. Not to do those rituals—to change—is frightening. The anxiety threatens to become unrestrained.
- *Resistance* to change is present in every task that the therapy undertakes. No matter how much patients want to ameliorate the problems the therapy plans to fix, they paradoxically resist every invitation to do so. Their opposition often is not a voluntary or even a conscious choice. A large part of therapeutic work is the continual effort to overcome some amount of resistance. When it threatens to stop or deflect the treatment, the entire focus of the therapy must shift to this effort, at least until resistance is diminished enough that the central therapeutic tasks can resume.
- The necessity of change increases the importance of the therapeutic contract, the agreement between therapist and patient about what behaviors should change, and how, together, they plan to change them. It is important that the focus of the work be actual behavioral change. Obvious as this sounds, it is not an automatic or a certain outcome of the therapy effort. Therapist and patient might agree, for instance, that the therapy should strive to provide the patient with greater self-knowledge or insight. If these accomplishments do not lead to some ameliorative behavioral change, the therapy will have been a failure.

BEHAVIOR

Behavior is another word for actions. How a patient behaves is reflected in the *actions* she or he takes. These actions, for example, might include the compulsive rituals noted earlier, a decrease in food intake in depression, or withdrawal during a psychotic episode. An action might be a so-cial response, such as not making eye contact when speaking to another person, or something done alone, such as binge eating. It could be trivial, such as the overuse of the word "like" ("I, like, told him I would, like, meet him, like, later"), or life-altering, such as the avoidance of close and trusting relationships. Insight, by contrast, might be an instrument of change, but it is not a behavior, and an insight, in itself, changes nothing.

- Thoughts are also behavior. One definition of thought is *trial action*: we think of what to do before we do it. A thought is also an action in itself, although perhaps an involuntary one (Don't picture a unicorn).
- Feelings are not behavior. Emotional responses are not under our control and cannot be *directly* affected by therapy. A change in be-havior, however, can alter the feeling associated with it. For instance,

  ➤ Arranging your face into a smiling expression will make the world around you seem more pleasant, even amusing.
  ➤ An expansive posture, in which you take up as much space as possible, can alter brain hormones and increase subjective feelings of confidence and power.
  ➤ For a clinical example of how behavior can affect emotion, we can once again cite the case of Elizabeth. Forcing herself into a phobic environment initially increased her anxiety but then, with repeti-tion, dispelled it.

POWER

The final characteristic of psychotherapy is the unequal distribution of *power*. As the therapist, your power is embodied in control of the time, the calendar, and the office environment. It is reflected in the disparity between the patient's required openness and vulnerability and your re-striction of personal information and speech. It is embodied in your deci-sions about interventions. Although the patient has the ultimate power—represented by the decision to continue the process or stop it and leave—the proximal power rests with you.

The patient might be expected to have "the power of the purse" through the threat of withholding payment. In our current health care environ-ment, however, this power is wielded primarily by third-party payers. These third parties may be

- Private, if the patient has purchased coverage out of pocket.
- Corporate, if health insurance is a benefit supplied by the employer.
- Governmental, through programs such as Medicaid and Medicare.

Third-party power distorts the therapy. Limitations and restrictions on service, price controls applied to fees, additional paperwork, delays in payment, and intrusive demands for information all force themselves between you and your patient and create nontherapeutic burdens that distract from therapy goals and may damage the working relationship. Third-party payers not only bias the balance of power; they can sabotage the entire therapy. Nevertheless, the patient usually pays some portion of the fee and thus holds some portion of this monetary power.

Even though patients have this potential economic power, however, what they can control is limited by your professional status. A professional can be hired but cannot be told what to do. You can hire a surgeon, for instance, but you cannot direct the operation. You can hire an accountant, but you cannot control the results of an audit. In the same way, the patient who hires you cannot control the therapy.

Because power is distributed unequally, then, the therapeutic relationship is *asymmetrical*. Some therapies—existential, for example—may aspire to a symmetrical relationship: two human beings meeting on an equal footing. This "equal relationship," however, only occurs (if it is achieved at all) within the therapeutic model. Otherwise, asymmetry prevails. You retain most of the power in the relationship, even if both parties choose to ignore it. For instance:

- The patient pays you.
- The encounter occurs only in a setting of your choosing, usually your office.
- Even a home visit session occurs only when and if you choose to make it.

An interesting slant on this power inequality is the *therapeutic paradox*.[7] This theory makes the exercise of power, as a feature of the therapeutic alliance, the central ameliorative force in the treatment. Change in the therapeutic context, according to Haley, results from the ordeal of the therapy under the guidance of a benevolent process, from which the patient can only escape by giving up the problematic behavior.

- Therapy is an ordeal because
    - ➤ It costs the patient money and time.
    - ➤ It provokes unpleasant emotions.

---

[7]Haley J: *Strategies of Psychotherapy.* New York, Grune & Stratton, 1963.

➢ Its procedures are sometimes humiliating, may appear punitive, and can be emotionally painful.

- Your benevolent stance, your half of the therapeutic alliance, is based on the patient's
  ➢ Request for help from you.
  ➢ Voluntary participation in the process.
  ➢ Appreciation of your healing intention and good will toward the patient.

In paradoxical therapy, you do not order the patient to forgo the symptoms of emotional dysfunction—that would be a direct exercise of power that the patient would reflexively oppose—but, until the patient "improves," the ordeal you impose will go on and on. Haley suggested that this mechanism is at the core of every therapeutic method, whether psychodynamic, cognitive-behavioral, or existential. The theory behind each method and the procedures by which that theory becomes a methodology are only variations on this basic scheme: a benevolent despot imposing a punishing ordeal in the service of positive therapeutic change.

The idea that you must exercise power over the patient may be an uncomfortable concept. The exercise of power can have negative implications. Power can be abused. Your role as healer may seem incompatible with exerting power over the very person the therapy is intended to help. Keep in mind that you will use that power to create a benefit for your patient and that the patient's participation is voluntary. The patient

- Chooses to employ you.
- Participates willingly in your program.
- Can leave at any time.

Beneficial asymmetric relationships are mirrored elsewhere in free societies:

- We place ourselves under the care of other health care providers in return for medical or surgical help.
- We cede power to the police in return for safety and public order.
- We give power to elected officials in return for their representation of our interests.

The same trade-offs occur with military volunteers, members of a sports team, use of an investment advisor, and so on. Your patients agree to give up power, temporarily, in order to acquire the benefits of the therapy: reduced dysphoria, symptom relief, a more satisfactory life.

These four components—transaction, change, behavior, power—together define the characteristics of psychotherapy. Taken as a whole, they specify a unique service. Table 2–7 summarizes the mechanisms and targets of these components.

TABLE 2–7. Psychotherapy components

Component	Mechanism	Target problem
Transaction	Communication: exchange of information (patient) for guidance (therapist)	Patient's editing and self-censorship
Change	Give up usual but ineffective coping style for new, more helpful strategies and beliefs	Resistance, direct and indirect, conscious and unconscious
Behavior	Decrease or forgo old (dysfunctional) behavior; increase or add new (adaptive) behavior	Homeostasis: tendency to maintain existing behavior despite its drawbacks
Power	Therapist gains from professional status, control of the environment, expert knowledge	Opposition based on drive for independence or overdependence

A Note About Cybertherapy

I have discussed psychotherapy as an activity between two persons. Online psychotherapy, in which the two participants communicate by video or by text (e-mail or chat programs), may select for patients who are uncomfortable in face-to-face meetings. Individuals feel less inhibited in this format and are able to reveal personal information with less embarrassment or fear of judgment. Online communication means that patients can review your statements more than once and increase their understanding of them. The reduced inhibition, along with affordability and the elimination of travel, can make this option more accessible and may result in a good outcome for patients who would otherwise be untreated.

Increasingly, however, a new alphanumeric entity joins the dyad. As part of the digital revolution, efforts are under way to develop more effective, reliable, widely applicable computer-based psychotherapy programs. Software therapy programs have been around for decades, beginning with ELIZA, an interactive program developed by Joseph Weizenbaum at the Massachusetts Institute of Technology on the basis of nondirective (Rogerian[8]) therapy.[9] Weizenbaum wanted to test whether a computer could communicate using natural language. It couldn't. Although some users reported useful interactions with ELIZA, others found it frustrating and dim-witted.

More recent programs, however, have been more successful. They use cognitive-behavioral protocols to help patients with depression, a variety of anxiety disorders, eating disorders, substance abuse problems, and others. The participation of a human therapist, at least to monitor and troubleshoot the process, appears necessary, but the therapist's involvement is reduced to perhaps one-fifth of the therapy time. The "therapist" can be a person trained for the program and not highly credentialed—in other words, not a professional. The program user, after all, does not know who is on the other side of the screen. Among other advantages, one "cybertherapist" can treat five patients in the same time that is required for a single, face-to-face therapy session.

The appeal of cybertherapy programs is obvious:

- Many parts of the world are too poor or too undeveloped to provide mental health services to large populations in need. A cheap alternative would provide care for millions in remote areas.
- Third-party payers, both corporate and government, for whom cost reduction is the highest priority and profit the overriding motive, would welcome a low-cost, machine-based alternative to human therapists. No doubt, some important development funding will come from these stakeholders.
- Patients can work some or all of the program from home, on their own timetables, reducing demand for office space and personnel. This expanded access would provide more services to more people while reducing overhead costs.

---

[8]See, for example, Rogers CR: *Client-Centered Therapy: Its Current Practice, Implications and Theory.* London, Constable, 1951.

[9]Weizenbaum J: "ELIZA—A Computer Program for the Study of Natural Language Communication Between Man and Machine." *Communications of the ACM* 9:36–45, 1966.

- Interaction with a computer reduces the stigma associated with mental health care. Patients who might avoid a mental health facility could be steered to programs based in primary care facilities or use home-based applications for greater privacy.
- Computer services can be enhanced by multimedia and scaled up without limit. Video and other enhancements may make programs more effective. Virtual reality and the use of therapist avatars may increase the illusion that the computer is human.

BUT IS IT PSYCHOTHERAPY?

I defined *psychotherapy* as a transactional method to change behavior within an asymmetrical power relationship. A computer-based psychotherapy program meets this definition, perhaps with the single caveat that the distribution of power shifts toward the patient. In many cases, the patient controls the time and place of treatment, as well as the frequency and intensity of the program's use. Unlike a face-to-face encounter, however, communication is limited to verbal messages entered or received on a screen. Nonverbal communication is diminished or completely absent. The "therapist," if human, may appear only as a face or head and shoulders, as would the patient. A text-based program loses even that. Although patients may "animate" the computer program and assign it such characteristics as benign regard and disinterested concern, the relationship never reaches the intensity or depth provided by a human therapist. The computer does have one advantage: it does not judge. As someone has observed, computers have no eyebrows.

CAN WE BE REPLACED BY COMPUTERS?

At present, these programs are at an early stage and have been limited to cognitive-behavioral protocols that lend themselves most readily to software algorithms. It seems *unlikely* that these programs could replace a psychodynamic or existential therapist because they lack the spontaneous interactive skills required, but "unlikely" in today's fast-moving world of technology does not mean "will never happen." Microsoft, for example, has demonstrated a new software that can recognize human emotions from facial expressions.

Imagine an onscreen animation better than what you now see in films and video games, so realistic that you cannot tell it from an onscreen human. This computer-generated avatar speaks in natural language with all the intuition and nuances of a human therapist. It responds not only to your words (no keyboard needed; it understands when you speak) but also your nonverbal communication. It chooses one of its programmed methodologies and guides you through its protocol. It senses resistance and deals with it until the program can resume. In fact, imagine that the cybertherapist is a humanoid robot. It looks like a person and has human facial expressions and a human voice. It even has eyebrows. Is this a realistic possibility?

During the Great War in Europe, 1914 to 1918—only a hundred years ago—the new technology was a propeller-driven biplane with a pilot who dropped crude bombs over the side of the cockpit. None of the combatants could imagine that today unmanned aerial vehicles (drones) would fly thousands of miles above the battlefield, able to examine it in such exquisite detail as to discern the chevrons on a soldier's sleeve. Or that drones could deliver high-explosive missiles with pinpoint accuracy against targets selected by an operator thousands of miles away using satellites in geosynchronous orbit. It is nearly as difficult for us to imagine that one hundred years from now, digital algorithms will mimic human intuition and empathy and use natural language to provide psychodynamic psychotherapy to a patient through a virtual reality interface. Nevertheless, if Moore's Law (computing power doubles every two years) holds true, then machines with the capacity to undertake complex interactions using future versions of artificial intelligence are *likely* to replace more and more of the functions now unique to human therapists.

Whether these programs ever reach parity with humans seems a far-off possibility—not in my lifetime and probably not in yours—but given the ongoing technological revolution, that parity cannot be ruled out. In the meantime, we need all the human therapists we can get.

General Types of Therapy

As I noted earlier, this book cannot cover the multiplicity of psychotherapies available to a therapist today. For the sake of later discussions, however, I will briefly review examples of the three general types of therapeutic modalities: exploratory, directive, and experiential.

EXPLORATORY

Exploratory approaches concentrate on elements from the past and the unrecognized or unconscious factors that influence current behavior. Psychodynamic psychotherapy, for instance, locates the patient's current symptoms in unresolved conflicts, often originating in early to middle childhood. "As the twig is bent, so grows the tree." This old adage captures that theory and also illustrates its widespread acceptance outside the mental health field as a basic truth of human development. Another model that illustrates this approach is a tower of blocks. Imagine that each phase of childhood development is a block. If the blocks are perfect cubes, meaning normal developmental experiences, the tower will remain stable as additional blocks are stacked on over time. If a block is misshapen, lower on one side than the other, indicating a flawed or failed transition, the added blocks will tilt more and more until the tower falls. These uneven blocks are childhood deficits and defects. The more deformed the blocks, the shakier the tower and the patient's mental health (Figure 2–2). This simple model, of course, presumes that a single childhood "event" can explain adult pathology. In fact, the child's developmental trauma would be better represented if the tower contained several misshapen blocks, reflecting the ongoing effects of an adverse environment, whose *cumulative* effect would determine later behavior.

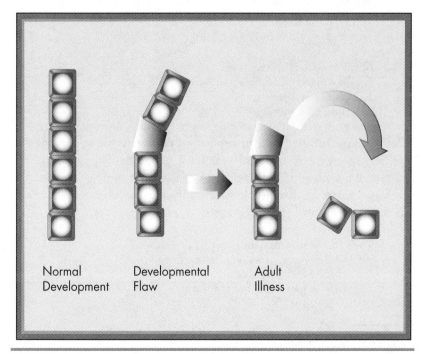

Normal Development

Developmental Flaw

Adult Illness

FIGURE 2–2. **Psychodynamic model.**

DIRECTIVE

Directive therapies originate in various psychological theories of learning, with the premise that current behavior represents an ingrained pattern of responses to past stresses and traumas. Cognitive-behavioral therapy (CBT), for example, focuses on learned maladaptive behavior as the cause of current symptoms. Past history is often considered irrelevant, except as it documents the antecedents of the target behavior and the reinforcing conditions that sustain it. Because CBT is based on the psychology of learning, it relies on psychological strategies that use new learning experiences to replace unwanted behaviors with more adaptive ones.

EXPERIENTIAL

Experiential therapies emphasize immediate experience, the direct encounter with the complexities of life. Existential therapy, for instance, tries to help the patient find meaning in life, especially when confronted with the uncomfortable idea that an individual life has none. As Leo Tolstoy asked as he contemplated suicide in his early fifties, "What meaning has life that death does not destroy?"[10] Or as Andrew Marvell put it[11]:

> But at my back I always hear
> Time's wingèd chariot hurrying near
> and yonder all before us lie
> deserts of vast eternity.

After we have fulfilled our biological imperative to procreate and disseminate our genetic material—after we produce offspring—life appears to have no other biological purpose, and, almost always, our death will leave no discernible or meaningful residue behind to mark our existence. From Thomas Gray[12]:

> The boast of heraldry, the pomp of power,
> And all that beauty, all that wealth e'er gave,
> Awaits alike the inevitable hour.
> The paths of glory lead but to the grave.

---

[10]A Confession, 1879–1880.

[11]"To His Coy Mistress," 1650.

[12]"Elegy Written in a Country Churchyard," 1751.

Philosophy and religion, two major efforts to counter the despair that contemplation of this reality usually produces, provide the underpinnings for this methodology.

A subset of these therapies includes those approaches that avoid "talk" in favor of actions, movement, and direct experience. Examples include art therapy and psychodrama.

Each of these three general groups contains a multitude of separate methodologies, and some try to bridge or combine two categories. Dialectical behavior therapy, a system designed to treat people with borderline personality disorder, for example, uses a combination of directive and experiential interventions. Table 2–8 summarizes the characteristics of the three general approaches to psychotherapy.

TABLE 2–8. General types of psychotherapy

	Exploratory	Directive	Experiential
Example	Psychodynamic psychotherapy	Cognitive-behavioral therapy	Existential therapy
Core explanation (myth)	Unresolved historical conflict	Learned maladaptive thinking	Search for meaning
Therapist's activity level	Low	High	Medium
Therapeutic focus	Remembered events	Current behavior	Human condition
Main therapeutic activity (ritual)	Interpretation	Instruction and guidance	Shared experience

Your commitment to one of these three approaches will be determined, in part, by your personal style.

- If you like to investigate past personal history and to study the effect of the past on the present, you will lean toward exploratory theories.
- If you prefer an active role, focused on current behavior, and like to educate and explain, you will be drawn to directive therapies.
- If you have a philosophical bent, want to avoid labeling, and are more comfortable with assisting patients than directing them, you will gravitate toward experiential therapies.

Whatever your preference, however, you will be more successful if you acquire competence in more than one therapy approach. Different patients will benefit from each of these three types of therapy. If you limit yourself to only a single type and discard the other two, your effectiveness will suffer. To illustrate the different styles, we can see how you might approach the same patient from each of the three conceptual systems.

Clinical Examples

Earlier in this chapter, we met Gregory, a 75-year-old man, ruminating about the end of his life. Gregory is a widower, having lost his wife, Carol, to cancer two years ago. He then retired from his law practice and looked forward to playing more golf, spending time with his children and grandchildren, and perhaps writing a novel based on one of his interesting cases. Instead, he began to lose interest in golf; his children, busy with their own lives, did not include him as he had hoped; and the novel remained unwritten. It is his third session.

PSYCHODYNAMIC PSYCHOTHERAPY

Gregory	I spent the whole day yesterday getting nothing done.
You	What did you want to accomplish?
Gregory	Well, first I thought I'd go to the driving range, but I couldn't work up any enthusiasm. My game's not getting any better. I might as well throw away my clubs. Then, I called my daughter but no answer. And I sat for a while thinking of a title for the book. Then, I had lunch, and afterward I fell asleep. The whole day just went on like that.
You	You sound angry.
Gregory	I am angry. It wasn't supposed to be this way.
You	How so?
Gregory	Carol and I, we had big plans. I'd retire and we'd travel the world. We were going to take cooking classes. She planned to learn golf.
You	So you're angry at Carol?

Gregory	What? I didn't say that. It wasn't her fault she got cancer. She didn't want to die.
You	If not Carol, who are you angry at?
Gregory	Fate. The Universe. I don't know.
You	That would make it easier, wouldn't it? Better to be mad at the universe than at Carol.
Gregory	Look, being mad at Carol just makes no sense. My mother always told me anger was like a poison in your mouth.
You	Is your mother still alive?
Gregory	No, she died a long time ago.
You	What was she like?
Gregory	She was…kind, caring…always proud of me.
You	Proud of you?
Gregory	Sure. You know, only son and all that.
You	Think back. Were you angry when your mother died?
Gregory	I don't…well, I had…. It's embarrassing. I guess to-day we'd call it road rage. A guy cut in front of me in bumper-to-bumper traffic. He was driving one of those little VW Bugs, and I was in a big, heavy car. A Jeep. I was furious. I pulled up to his rear bumper and just pushed him off the road.
You	And this was after your mother died?
Gregory	The day after the funeral.
You	So that's twice. Someone close to you dies and you're angry.

This session has followed a typical process for psychodynamic therapy, which usually involves four steps:

1. Identification: Gregory is angry.
2. Clarification: He is angry at Carol, who frustrated his retirement plans when she died.
3. Interpretation: He avoids anger at Carol by blaming Fate.
4. Working through: His mother's death was also followed by anger.

The psychodynamic premise is: Gregory is unable to move forward in his life because of his unacknowledged anger at his dead wife.

COGNITIVE-BEHAVIORAL THERAPY

Gregory	I spent the whole day yesterday getting nothing done.
You	What did you want to accomplish?
Gregory	Well, first I thought I'd go to the driving range, but I couldn't work up any enthusiasm. My game's not getting any better. I might as well throw away my clubs. Then, I called my daughter but no answer. And I sat for a while thinking of a title for the book. Then, I had lunch, and afterward I fell asleep. The whole day just went on like that.
You	So then you had three things you wanted to do, but none of them worked out.
Gregory	That's right. The day was a complete and total waste.
You	OK, but let's go over what you said about yesterday. What about lunch? Did you enjoy your meal?
Gregory	I did.
You	And how about your nap? Did you feel refreshed when you woke up?
Gregory	I felt rested.
You	So both of those were positive events. You enjoyed your food while you satisfied your hunger, and you caught up on your rest.
Gregory	True, but those were minor. Just bodily functions. They weren't the important things.
You	Do you remember we talked last time about automatic thoughts?
Gregory	Yes.
You	I want you to think back. What went through your mind when you decided not to go out? Or when your daughter didn't answer the phone?

Gregory	(*thinks for a moment*) Well, I remember thinking nothing ever works out for me. That's what I thought. Because it's true.
You	What did you feel when you had that thought, "Nothing ever works out for me"?
Gregory	I felt angry. Frustrated and angry, and then I felt sad. I didn't have the energy to do anything, so I took a nap.
You	When you decided the day was a complete and total waste, that was a negative overgeneralization, a totally negative judgment. There were three things that didn't work out yesterday, but there were also two positive things. And because of your automatic thought, you didn't try any more. The thought made you angry, and then the sadness made you give up.
Gregory	Well, I can't disagree with that, but how does that help me?
You	I think we've identified something we can work on: when your plans don't pan out, you conclude everything is useless. That negative idea—nothing ever works out—leads you to the next idea: there's no use trying. For instance, you don't know that working on your golf swing wouldn't have helped your game. Maybe it would have. And if you'd called your daughter later, when she was home, you might have been able to arrange the visit you wanted to make. You would have seen her and the grandchildren after all. Instead, you gave up because that thought—nothing ever works out—kept you from trying. That made it a self-fulfilling prophesy. Nothing will ever work out because you don't try to make it happen.
Gregory	Maybe you're right, but what should I do about it? I can't help the way I think.
You	Actually, you can. Experience shows that if you change your behavior, your negative thinking will

decrease. Before you leave today, I'll give you some reading to do, and we'll go over it next time. What I'd also like you to do: Between now and our next session, I'd like you to keep a daily log of your activities. For each day, keep a running account of your plans and how they work out. Just jot them down: I had breakfast, I watched the news, I played golf. Be sure you also note what you didn't do: I wanted to play golf, but it was raining. I wanted to write my first chapter, but I couldn't see how to start. Try to identify what goes through your mind and what you're feeling at that moment and what you do, and write that down as well.

Gregory   I can do that.

You   Good. Let's see how many things work out and how many don't. Next week we'll go over the list and decide how big a problem it is. We'll explore whether negative thinking is an important source of your problem. If it is, I can suggest some strategies to combat it.

Notice how much more talking you did in this CBT session than you did in the psychodynamic interview. You educated Gregory about automatic thoughts[13] and gave him reading material to reinforce the idea (sometimes called *bibliotherapy*). Notice also that you did not explore any possible connections between his anger and his wife's death or his earlier anger after his mother died. Those potential past connections were not relevant to your treatment plan. Instead, you identified an automatic thought and explained the impact it was having on Gregory's behavior. Then, you assigned him homework as part of a beginning plan of corrective action. The premise is that automatic thoughts can be identified, and the patient can learn to modify them. A learned habit of negative overgeneralization can be corrected by training the patient how to assess challenges more realistically and with alternative expectations.

---

[13]*Automatic thoughts* are critical self-judgments that appear as apparently spontaneous ideas. They are associated with dysphoric feelings, such as sadness, and dysfunctional behavior, such as giving up. They reflect long-held, destructive attitudes and assumptions that originate in negative core beliefs.

EXISTENTIAL PSYCHOTHERAPY

Gregory	I spent the whole day yesterday getting nothing done.
You	What did you want to accomplish?
Gregory	Well, first I thought I'd go to the driving range, but I couldn't work up any enthusiasm. My game's not getting any better. I might as well throw away my clubs. Then, I called my daughter but no answer. And I sat for a while thinking of a title for the book. Then, I had lunch, and afterward I fell asleep. The whole day just went on like that.
You	You found those events very frustrating.
Gregory	A lot of my days have been like that. I get up full of good intentions and I think I'm going to do something, you know. I mean, I make these plans and somehow they don't work out for me. My life is slipping away. How many days do I have left? The clock is ticking, ticking. (*He starts to cry.*) Pretty soon it'll be all over, and what a waste! I thought I'd be happier when I finished working. I didn't like law practice. So many problems, always under pressure. Pressure to keep my hours up. I thought when my time was my own, and I didn't need to stay on the treadmill just to stay even, that I'd be busy with my own stuff. Me and Carol. But then she died and I retired anyway. But it's no good without her.
You	You miss her a lot.
Gregory	I really do. I mean, it wasn't a perfect marriage, but I think we had something good. And now, even a couple of years later I still want to tell her things. Something will happen, or I'll come across some interesting news item, and before I realize it I'm rehearsing in my mind how I'm going to tell her about it. [*He stares ahead for a few moments in silence.*] We had plans. We wanted to travel, all over, other countries. We were going to China, India. Now it's all for shit.

You	Without her, your plans have lost their meaning.
Gregory	That's right. I have no direction. That's what my life needs now.
You	Don't we all feel that way? I know I do at times. But who's responsible for it? It can't be Carol. She's gone. Can it be your children? Are they responsible?
Gregory	The children? Of course not. They're busy. They have their own lives. I'm all alone now, so I guess I'm responsible.
You	Perhaps you've been avoiding that responsibility, and that's why you feel helpless.
Gregory	But I *could* make more of an effort. I know that. [*He paces the room.*] I think I will. I think I'll try to set up something on a regular basis with them. Maybe take them out to dinner. Maybe a round of golf. My son-in-law plays, and I taught my daughter the game. She was pretty good back when she was single. My son's not a golfer, but I know he likes music. I could get some concert tickets. It would make Carol happy, knowing the family was still getting together.
You	But Carol's dead. Can you make her happy?
Gregory	I know, I know. All right, it would make me feel better. Doing it for Carol.... I'd honor her memory, but I'd be the one to benefit.
You	Our time is up. We have to stop.

In this existential therapy example, you say the least of the three illustrations. Instead of interpreting Gregory's ideas, you often simply restate what he feels using different wording. Again, it is not Gregory's anger that is central to the work, but rather his anxiety about how to manage the rest of his life, which he recognizes as limited. You focus on the here-and-now issues, specifically, the patient's need to confront the meaninglessness of his life and the way he avoids taking responsibility for it. You briefly disclose your own feelings as a way to let Gregory know he is dealing with problems common to everyone. Your effort to "be with" Gregory has apparently encouraged him to think through what is important to his life right now, and he has made a plan to act on this conclusion.

Final Thoughts

The definition of psychotherapy offered here—a transactional method to change problem behaviors through an asymmetric power relationship—does not establish a clear line of separation between psychotherapy and all other types of interpersonal discourse. At the margins, some activities may share its characteristics and yet not be "psychotherapy." As an example, consider sports psychology. The sports psychologist is a professional who helps athletes attain optimal performance and wellbeing using knowledge drawn from biomechanics and physiology and kinesiology, in addition to psychology. At times, the two might even focus on such mental health issues as depression, substance abuse, or eating disorders. All the components of the definition are present, but the work of the sports psychologist is not usually considered psychotherapy. Perhaps we should picture the discipline of psychotherapy as a series of ripples widening out from a stone dropped into a pond: strong, dense ripples at the center, weakening as they spread outward, finally fading into still water. Some undertakings are clearly psychotherapy, but at the edges it may be hard to tell when therapy merges into other areas of human interaction. Like Supreme Court Justice Potter Stewart said of pornography, we cannot completely define it, but we know it when we see it.

A group of core principles underlies every school of psychotherapy, and each of them builds on these principles, adding a superstructure of methods and procedures. In this way, each school more or less codifies its methodology. In your actual day-to-day work with specific patients, you must often improvise, be flexible, apply ideas learned from the hands-on experience with previous patients, and adapt whatever methodology you usually follow to the needs of a particular patient. In a high-tech world, psychotherapy remains low tech. Although computer programs can mimic psychotherapy, and even show some success, they are not as empathic, as nuanced, as effective as we human therapists. "Talk therapy" has modest but real benefits. Not the instant fix associated with modern technology and medical miracles, but benefits that can be long-lasting, even permanent. It gives people a sense of agency and control, active mastery rather than passive reception of treatments administered by others

The varieties of psychotherapy form a spectrum. At one end are the didactic protocols set up for selected target symptoms. At the other end, psychotherapy shades into philosophy, spirituality, or quasi-religion.

- Some of us are drawn to the protocols of targeted therapies. They offer a clear path with direction and purpose and a high likelihood of success within narrowly defined parameters. At this end of the spectrum lies the hope of following the medical paradigm: examine, test, diagnose, and treat.
- Some of us are intrigued by longitudinal causation: how does past experience shape the present? This middle ground seeks to provide relief from the mixture of problems identified by a patient with a unique life story.
- Some of us respond to the spiritual lure of self-actualization offered by the search for meaning and the patient's true self. Underlying the spiritual end is the conviction that the therapeutic relationship is a pathway to enlightenment that brings meaning to a patient's life.

Key Points

- Every culture has evolved a healing paradigm that involves a designated therapist, a special setting, a rationale or theory, and a specified activity that together will enable a patient to recover from emotional, behavioral, and social dysfunction.

- All of the multitude of psychotherapies share certain core characteristics.

- The core features include the placebo response and nonspecific factors, such as the evocation of strong emotion.

- All psychotherapeutic improvement involves affective experience, cognitive mastery, and behavioral regulation.

- Psychotherapy can be defined as a transactional process designed to change behavior through the exercise of interpersonal power in an asymmetric relationship.

- Computer-based psychotherapy protocols are currently of limited application and will likely improve, but they are far from being able to supplant human therapists.

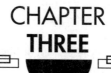

CHAPTER
THREE

What Is the Psychotherapy Relationship?

Je le pansai, Dieu le guérit.
(I bandaged him, God healed him.)

Ambroise Paré, famed 16th-century battlefield physician, on being praised for his surgical skill

In theory, there's no difference between theory and practice. In practice, there is.

Yogi Berra

Introduction

In the last chapter, I reviewed the healing forces that provide a foundation for any individual psychotherapy. In this chapter, I discuss the mechanism through which those forces are brought to bear. A fish in the water does not feel wet: although the water provides buoyancy, oxygen, support, and shelter, it is simply the medium in which the fish moves. In the same way, the psychotherapy participants may be unaware of the therapeutic milieu in which they operate, the interpersonal and environmental factors that support the healing process. Yet these factors are crucial to psychotherapeutic success. They are subsumed under the general heading of the psychotherapy relationship, but it is useful to examine its component elements. To be successful, you must pay as much attention to the milieu as you do to your specific therapeutic modality.

Definition

The *psychotherapy relationship* is a temporary association between a mental health professional and a person who acknowledges the need for improvement or healing in some personal aspect of life.[1] These two people, a dyad, meet together for reciprocal benefit:

- For you, the exercise of professional skills in return for payment.
- For the patient, the investment of time, money, and emotion in return for the amelioration of his or her behavioral difficulties.

In individual psychotherapy, the relationship has certain special and unique characteristics:

- The two people are unrelated.
- They only meet under a predetermined set of conditions involving
  - ➤ An appointment: based on an agreed time,
  - ➤ A session: based on the length of time,
  - ➤ A setting: usually your office, and
  - ➤ A payment, although funds are often from some third party.
- The content of their meeting remains confidential and even, to a limited extent, enjoys a legal privilege.
- At some point, their relationship ends.

Nature of a Psychotherapy Relationship

Psychotherapy is sometimes criticized as being only purchased friendship, notwithstanding that "paid friendship" is an oxymoron. To see why this condescending attitude is untrue, we can turn to Greek philosophy. In his *Nicomachean Ethics*, Aristotle examines the concept of friendship at length. I paraphrase—and simplify—his definition as a relationship with three characteristics:

- It entails mutual respect.
- It occurs between equals.
- It persists over a long period of time.

A comparison of psychotherapy and friendship according to this definition highlights the differences (Table 3–1):

---

[1]An *involuntary* psychotherapy association, such as court-mandated treatment, often lacks this essential component and is unlikely to be successful.

TABLE 3–1. Aristotelian friendship versus psychotherapy

Quality	Friendship	Psychotherapy
Mutual respect	Yes: reciprocated good opinion	No: unbalanced because of patient deficits or conflicts
Between equals	Yes: coequal partners	No: asymmetric, unequal power
Long time period	Yes: the longer, the better	No: unusual, undesirable

1. "Mutual respect," in this context, means the recognition by each person of "the good" in the other. Because the regard is "mutual," each has the same positive assessment of the other person. A statement more relevant to a therapy relationship is that in friendship both accept the other "as is" and do not require either to change. The high value they place on the other person's qualities represents a reciprocal and equivalent balance. In contrast, a psychotherapy relationship assumes an imbalance: the patient has fallen short of "the good," is dysfunctional in some particulars, and you, the therapist, are presumed to be free of this dysfunction. This inequality skews the "respect" each of you has for the other. The patient must consider you a competent, caring professional or the therapy will be ineffective. You, while respectful of the patient in other areas, must acknowledge that emotional problems prevent the patient from fully realizing normal function.

2. The requirement of "between equals" is also absent. As I noted in the previous chapter, the balance of power in the psychotherapy relationship is asymmetrical, and therefore equality is not possible or desirable.

3. "Over a long period of time" is not typical; most therapies are relatively short. Although some might extend over many years, the usual length of treatment is in the range of a dozen or so weekly sessions. Even a year's worth of weekly therapy is, on average, unusual. Patients who come less frequently may continue for longer, but as the time between sessions lengthens, the continuity and effectiveness of the treatment are apt to diminish. In short, when conducted over a long period of time, psychotherapy is increasingly less likely to produce the desired outcome. Some wag has said that it is the only treatment that when it fails to work, the prescription is for more of it.

So, if psychotherapy is not friendship, what features does it share with other dyads? How do these dyads differ from psychotherapy, and what do they have in common (Table 3–2)?

- *Teacher-student.* Although therapy is, in part, an educational process, it is more concerned with changing behavior than with inculcating new facts.
- *Employer-employee.* The relationship is similar in that the therapist does sometimes assign work, but it is different because the patient is not paid for the work.
- *Salesperson-customer.* Persuasion is part of the therapist's job, but the patient pays the therapist even if there is "no sale."
- *Parent-child.* The therapist functions a little like a parent in guiding and caring for the patient, but the therapist is not responsible for the patient and provides no material support.
- *Physician-patient.* Again, there is similarity in the caretaking aspect of the therapy and the therapist's "prescription" of healing measures, but the physician expects compliance, whereas the therapist looks for collaborative cooperation.

Relationship Elements

The psychotherapy relationship, like Caesar's Gaul, is divided into three parts.[2]

Psychoanalytic descriptions of this relationship emphasize the transference-countertransference component,[3] along with the working alliance and the real relationship. In psychoanalysis, the transference-countertransference phenomenon is the main focus of treatment. In other therapies, it is dealt with as an impediment to the therapy but not as its major concern.

A somewhat different version of the tripartite nature of the psychotherapy relationship has evolved as other methodologies have devel-

---

[2]*The Gallic Wars* by Julius Caesar: "*Gallia est omnis divisa in partes tres.*"

[3]*Transference* refers to the projection onto the therapist of feelings, attitudes, expectations, and hopes that the patient experienced in the past, usually with parents but also with other significant childhood connections, such as teachers or, later on, with romantic partners. The transference distorts the patient's view of the therapist and can thereby disrupt the progress of treatment. *Countertransference* is the same phenomenon when it happens instead to the therapist. It has the same consequences for the therapy.

TABLE 3–2. Other dyads: similarities and differences

Therapist=	Patient=	Alike	Different
Teacher	Student	Education, facts	Behavioral change
Employer	Employee	Assigning work	No payment
Salesperson	Customer	Persuasion	Paid if no sale
Parent	Child	Caretaker, guide	Not responsible
Physician	Patient	Effort to heal	Collaboration, not compliance

oped. In this newer classification, transference and countertransference are included in the operational portion of the triad.

The three divisions, in this broader definition, are

1. *The real relationship,* the administrative, nontherapeutic dealings between you and the patient.
2. *The therapeutic alliance,* the collaborative, working partnership, independent of the therapeutic modality selected.
3. *The operational plan,* the desired outcome of the treatment, including the goals, methodologies, and techniques employed to reach it.

The real relationship is the smallest piece. The therapeutic alliance and the operational plan together make up the bulk of the therapy relationship. Although I make sharp delineations among them for the purpose of discussion, in the course of treatment the boundaries are blurred and sometimes overlap.

The balance of these three elements changes as therapy proceeds (Figure 3–1). At the beginning, before the treatment plan is implemented, the therapeutic alliance is almost the entire relationship. As the therapy proceeds, the operational plan, the "business" of the therapy, claims a larger share of it, and the alliance shrinks accordingly. The goodwill and cooperation that the alliance generated are reduced by the stress of the therapy on the patient. In this sense, the patient is willing to undergo the ordeal of the therapy not only because of its promise of healing but also because the alliance supports it. By building the alliance at the beginning of treatment, you accrue a kind of credit or capital that is then expended on the operational plan. As the therapy nears termination, when most of the problems have been addressed, the alliance again becomes stronger and will support the painful process leading to termination.

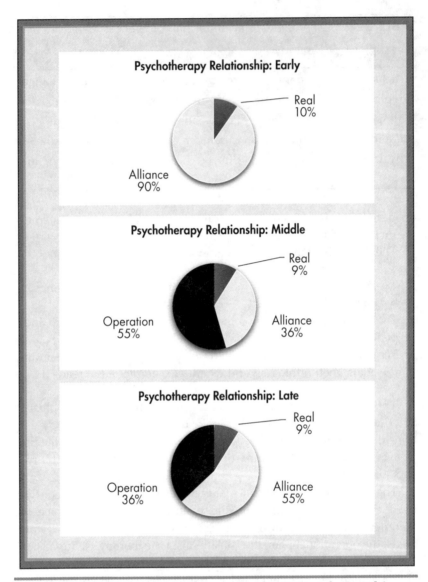

FIGURE 3–1.   Progression of psychotherapy relationship.

The meanings of the three parts are somewhat different from the psychoanalytic designations and require further explanation. Table 3–3 compares the elements of psychoanalytic and generic psychotherapies.

TABLE 3–3. Comparison of psychotherapy relationships

Psychoanalytic psychotherapy	Generic psychotherapy
Real relationship	Real relationship
Working alliance	Therapeutic alliance
Transference-countertransference	Operational plan

THE REAL RELATIONSHIP

The real relationship acknowledges the common humanity of both parties. Apart from your roles as patient and therapist, you both have undistorted perceptions that allow authentic appreciation of each other as individuals you can like, trust, and value. You recognize that you are ordinary persons who have other social roles and responsibilities. The patient knows that you

- Are paid for the work.
- Have other patients.
- Go home at the end of the day.
- Have a separate life outside the office.

You expect that the patient will

- Keep all appointments or give adequate notice.
- Arrive on time and leave when the session ends.
- Cooperate with whatever administrative arrangements are required.
- Pay bills in a timely fashion.
- Respect the office environment.

These aspects of the real relationship create expectations that are usually met, but when they are not, their failure impedes the therapeutic alliance and disrupts or diverts the operational plan.

Examples

The real relationship is usually unacknowledged. To illustrate, we can look outside the therapy office for examples from public life. In public places, like a street or an elevator, we ignore others and do not recognize that we share any common bonds. If someone acts outside this role, however, others will quickly respond. Aspects of the real relationship can be found in the way our separate behavior gives way to personal connection when circumstances change. Here are two small examples:

- I sneeze on a public street and receive a "God bless you" from a complete stranger who happens to be passing. My sneeze briefly changes our nonrelationship, allowing us to transcend our situational roles to let a real relationship emerge, even if it was only an effort to protect me from the nonexistent plague.[4] In our real relationship, we share some common characteristics; for example, we are both adults, both males, both pedestrians traveling to a destination. In the same way, if I sneeze during the session, my patient is likely to respond with a "God bless you," and I with "Thank you," after which we resume whatever discussion was in progress. The common cultural quirk transcends the situational role.
- Two people are ascending in an elevator. While it rises, our social custom requires that we stand apart, eyes front, not speaking. If I change the expectation, however, with some bland remark ("This elevator is really slow!"), the other person will drop the indifferent role and begin a friendly conversation about my topic. In a therapy session, the patient may be locked in a battle of wills, but if I point out that his wallet has fallen to the floor, he will (usually) pause in his diatribe, retrieve his wallet, make a neutral remark and thank me, then return to his topic. The real relationship emerges briefly from its place in the background.

Absent psychotic ideation, the patient will always recognize the real relationship. It serves to anchor the therapy relationship in social custom. You occupy the role of healer, the patient that of sufferer. Society sanctions your meeting in this context. Like fish unaware of the water in which they swim, we do not think about this context. It simply exists.

Real Relationship Problems

Problems occur in therapy when either the therapeutic alliance or the operational plan (through some consequence of the methodology) begins to encroach on the neutral territory of the real relationship. A common manifestation of this blurring is a payment problem: the patient is late paying the bill, even the smaller copay amount, then skips payment on the next bill, and so on. The unpaid balance begins to add up. The

---

[4]Pope Gregory the Great (540–604 A.D.) supposedly instituted this blessing to protect passersby from contracting bubonic plague from the person who sneezed.

patient is now "acting out"[5] a conflict with either you or the therapy. The use of a supposedly neutral area to express the conflict also protects the patient from disclosure and its imagined consequences. ("I forgot my checkbook" rather than "I'm too angry this week to pay you.") In addition, the patient has exercised one of the few powers remaining in the asymmetrical relationship: the power of the purse. You may be concerned by the deterioration in the real relationship and angry that the acting out threatens a loss of income, but you may be reluctant to raise a seeming "reality" matter as a behavioral problem. You may also feel that bringing up the patient's debt will make you seem materialistic or uncaring, more interested in your income than the patient's problems. In other words, you worry that you may damage your professional image and therefore the therapeutic alliance. Although you may see no direct opening to solve the problem, the only solution to this dilemma is to address it directly and discuss it as a therapy issue.

As an illustration, imagine my patient has a $20 copay but has not paid it for three consecutive weeks. At the beginning of the fourth session, I bring it up.

Me	Before we start today, I want to discuss your bill. You haven't made a payment in the last three weeks.
Patient	(*sneers*) Don't worry. You'll get your money.
Me	From your tone of voice, it sounds like you resent my asking about it. Should I not have brought it up?
Patient	Well, it's not like my twenty bucks is a big problem. What's it going to mean? You can't get gas for your car? Your kids won't eat this week?

> *So far, the patient keeps the discussion in the real relationship. Instead of saying he is angry at me, he angrily refers to my (presumed) real life: I drive a car; I have a family. In order to refocus the issue as a therapy problem, I ignore the content of his statement and identify the affect. And by the way, it's sixty bucks.*

Me	I think you're feeling angry with me. Why don't we discuss what that's all about?

---

[5]The patient's upset is expressed indirectly, "acted out" through behavior, rather than communicated directly in words and feelings, in the session.

| Patient | I'm not angry. I am a little annoyed. I'm worried about losing my job and you don't seem to care. If I get fired, I'm going to need the twenty dollars more than you. |

What this exchange shows is that not paying his fee allows this man to act out a complex set of feelings:

- I was not showing him the concern he merited.
- I could not appreciate his worry because I was well off financially while his income was at risk.
- I was indifferent to the fact that he needed the money more than (he supposes) I did.
- I was selfishly depriving him of necessities like fuel and food.
- I should not charge him the full fee.

Any of these issues could prove worthwhile in his therapy. Whatever value these psychodynamic considerations might have, of course, I still want him to bring his payments up to date. Even if I were in a salaried position, and not directly affected by his nonpayment, I would, nevertheless, want to discuss the unpaid clinic fee as an important therapy issue.

A common real relationship condition is that many therapists will charge for missed sessions, especially if it happens without adequate notice. As another illustration of the intrusion of therapy issues, a patient of mine (a lawyer, naturally) argued that if he had to pay for a missed session, it was still his time, and he was entitled to "sublet" it to somebody else. When I asked who would he get to buy the time from him, he could not identify anyone. This exchange led to a useful discussion of his social isolation and related issues.

Other problems acted out in the real relationship include

- Late arrivals for appointments (usually, progressively later each time).
- Canceled appointments.
- Excessive use of the telephone or other communications outside the office, designed to control the therapist's time and to increase contact with the therapist beyond the scheduled appointments.
- Boundary violations, including approaching the therapist away from the office.
- Bringing another person, unannounced, to the session.

Again, the solution is to acknowledge that the problem is not a part of the real relationship but has now moved into the therapy work and to confront it as a therapy issue. The patient may try to assert that the behavior is "real" and beyond normal control ("I was feeling suicidal," "Traffic was heavy"), but this defense must be questioned. Handled correctly, the resulting discussion will advance the therapy, both because it removes a growing problem and because it will generate new material.

As Figure 3–1 indicates, the real relationship constitutes a small but constant element of the psychotherapy.

Patient Records

An important aspect of the real relationship is the patient record. While the record is part of the administrative portion of the relationship—on a par with billing information and the appointment log—it has implications and risks for both therapist and patient. A patient record is a legal document, with all that implies. It is subject to subpoena in any legal proceeding, such as a malpractice claim or a billing dispute. Under certain circumstances, it is available to the patient. Prudence dictates that you record the minimum necessary information in your "official" patient record.

Today, the patient record is likely to be electronic and therefore subject to distribution that you or the patient does not intend it to have. For example, a diagnosis submitted with an insurance claim can be promulgated throughout all offices the patient visits and into any records that have contact with this insurance database. Given the continuing stigma attached to mental illness, a psychiatric diagnosis may prejudice another provider in ways that disadvantage your patient. The electronic health record (EHR) is hailed as a way to integrate and coordinate patient care among all providers, but less attention has been paid to its effect on privacy and confidentiality. Patients can exercise control over their medical histories only with great difficulty, and most do not even try. Think of your own health record. Does your dermatologist really need to know what you tell your gynecologist? Does the doctor you see for an earache really need to know that you had a urinary tract infection? Shared *irrelevant* medical information does not enhance the quality of care, but it does degrade patient privacy. Recognition that the information is not secure may inhibit a patient from reporting something important to the doctor in the consulting room.

In my view, the EHR is a clear and present danger to privacy and confidentiality. Once your entries are online and shared with other providers, they are vulnerable, out of your control, subject to theft by malicious, unauthorized access ("hacking"),[6] and, of more immediate threat, available for gossip by anyone who might know the patient (supposedly, we are all connected by "six degrees of separation") and subject to careless, indifferent, or mischievous handling, such as by another provider's medical staff.

Today, because of mobile and internet technology, every aspect of our lives is subject to data collection and digital scrutiny. Google, Facebook, and a host of other companies, large and small, give us "free" programs in return for access to everything we do on their Web sites. Our photos, texts, purchases, locations—our most private problems—are saved, stored, aggregated, and analyzed to be monetized for profit. Data brokers buy up and sell every detail of our technology-exposed lives. Not only do these companies ferret out our data, they use complex algorithms to predict what we will do next. These algorithmic invasions reveal not only personal private information in general, but they pinpoint our health-related activities as well. As one example, a woman who visits her gynecologist (according to her calendar app) and later browses in a Babies"R"Us store (as revealed by her mobile phone location) will be targeted, thanks to the marketer's algorithm, with advertising for products related to pregnancy and infant care. This assault on patient privacy means that anything you record in an online data system, like the EHR, will be at risk. The same caveat applies to e-mails, text messaging, and any other online resource. These vulnerabilities suggest you should record only the minimum, legally necessary data in the EHR and *expect* that your patient's privacy will be violated, although you and the patient may not ever know that it happened.

Another concern is legal liability. We live in a litigious society. If you are the subject of a legal proceeding, the "evidence" will rely to a large degree on what you have documented in your own records. Those records, however, also serve as your best defense, and better still is that you have complete control over what goes into them. (You must have a record. An absence of the record leaves you with no defense.) If a legal problem does arise, where you anticipate an order for your records to be produced, do not alter them, not by a single letter. If you are later required to give testimony about the case, you cannot be held responsible for any more than you can document; that is, no more than is in your patient record.

---

[6]The latest reporting shows that the prevalence of unauthorized, malicious access of EHRs is more than 20 *million*, and those are only the instances where it was actually discovered.

The minimum information recorded should include

- Date of service.
- Any new diagnosis.
- Any specific recommendations.
- Any suicidal or homicidal ideation expressed in the session.
- Your response to either of those threats.
- Any medication prescribed and instructions to patient about taking it.
- Your next session, either the date or the interval.

In other words, you should include data that specifically document your care of the patient in that session. Anything more than these facts can place you at risk. Ask yourself, "Would I want my patient to read these words? Would I want to hear them read out in a court of law?"

The official patient record is not your journal or diary. Avoid writing your opinion, your criticism, or your speculations. Official records should not be used as memory aids. If you need a set of notes to help you recall and manage your previous sessions, write a separate set of "process notes." File them separately from the patient record, and in written rather than electronic form. Destroy them when no longer needed and, if not before, then after the patient leaves treatment.

Since you should only rarely refer to written notes in front of the patient, the better habit is to train yourself to recall what you need. With practice, you can develop your associative memory to supply the history. While you may not remember everything *between* sessions, you will find that seeing and hearing the patient in front of you the next time will stimulate your memory to supply what you need. And, of course, you can always ask the patient to remind you.

Finally, you should usually not take notes during a session. The image of the therapist with a notebook in one hand and a pen in the other is a relic of the early psychoanalyst, sitting behind the couch, writing everything down. In modern therapy, taking notes (especially on some type of computer tablet or laptop) erects a barrier between you and your patient. It projects an image of detachment and treats the patient as a specimen.[7] These connotations can damage the therapeutic alliance. Learn

---

[7]Medical professionals face increasing competition between their patients and the EHR. Every consultation and exam room now has a computer. Their attention must be divided as they focus on the screen, enter patient data, and ignore the patient. For a therapist, this three-way relationship would be even more undesirable.

to rely on your memory and have confidence that you will retain important information. Only in the rare instance where you *want* to maintain distance, can note taking be a useful technique.

Patient Gifts

A gift from a patient is an infrequent, perhaps even rare, occurrence. After all, in the real relationship, the patient understands that you are compensated for your work. Gift giving, however, implies something extra, including not only its cost but also the time and effort to acquire the gift and the patient's recognition of it as something personal for you. Therapy work is hard and its procedures are an ordeal, so within the therapy itself, a gift would seem to be out of place.

The gift's possible meaning can be as

- A sincere appreciation.
- A bribe.
- A symbolic gesture.

If the gift is appropriate—if its value is not excessive, if the object is not extravagant, and if it is offered in context; that is, in relation to some therapy event or near the end of the work—it should be treated as a transaction within the real relationship. In short, accept the gift with thanks. The patient's accompanying explanation may shed further light on the motives behind the gesture, but most of the time this unusual act is simply to express appreciation for the help you have provided. Not to accept a gift will be felt as a rejection and will risk damaging not only the real relationship but also the therapeutic alliance.

That being said, you cannot help wondering about it.

- Why *this* gift?
- What is its message?
- Why now?

In the context of the therapy work of the moment, it may strike you as a bribe or even a symbolic gesture. You should still accept an appropriate gift, even if you intend to discuss it. Perhaps it is consistent with other aspects of the therapy; for example, a positive transference. If so, it can become fair game for raising questions, if not at the time the gift is given, then at some later point when a related issue comes up. On that occasion, you may carefully explore some aspect of it that is of a piece with the regular issues of the therapy. Since you have already accepted the gift, the discussion will be less of a blow to the patient.

THE THERAPEUTIC ALLIANCE

The therapeutic alliance is the shared assumption that no matter what emotions are stirred or what distortions are introduced by the progress of therapy, no matter how rough the going gets, the two participants are committed to a collaboration whose goal is to help the patient overcome whatever difficulties initiated their coming together. This "working association" may be the most significant portion of the psychotherapy relationship. It is formed by the combined contributions of both you and the patient (Table 3–4).

TABLE 3–4. Contributions to the therapeutic alliance

Source	Contribution	Features
Therapist	Personal attributes	Warmth, sincerity, flexibility, confidence, openness, tolerance, integrity, concern for the patient
	Professional presentation	Appropriate clothing, grooming, demeanor
	Abilities and skills	Empathy, knowledge, methodological expertise
Patient	Personal attributes	Emotional intelligence, mental status, ability to trust, maintenance of boundaries, motivation for treatment, prior therapy
	Therapy attitudes	Motivation for change, honest participation, acceptance of therapeutic rationale and process, respect for therapist, hopeful expectation
Setting	Safe environment	Protection of privacy (soundproofing, records)
	Professional design	Furnishings, décor
	Facilitating milieu	Seating, lighting

The Therapist's Contribution

You contribute not only the expectation of success inherent in your social role of healer but also a number of personal attributes:

- *Warmth*. This quality is conveyed by your genuine interest in your patient, both as a fellow human being and as someone placed under your care.
- *Sensitivity*. You demonstrate this skill by your ability to read the immediate situation, a combination of close observation and intuitive recognition of the dynamics of what you observe.
- *Flexibility*. As the therapy manager, you are willing and able to adapt to new developments with the creativity to abandon ineffective efforts in order to try new approaches.
- *Confidence*. When you know what you are doing, your expertise and experience will be in evidence and will encourage your patient.
- *Openness*. A straightforward attitude and a willingness to acknowledge mistakes and to correct your work as needed will create an atmosphere of trust and cooperation between you and your patient.
- *Tolerance*. Your refusal to make judgments, to voice criticisms, or to coerce your patient—your unconditional positive regard[8]—will help him or her to confide sensitive information and to reveal difficult emotions.
- *Integrity*. Your clear commitment to your patient and to the therapeutic process, and only to them, will reassure your patient and build trust in the relationship.
- *Concern for the whole person*. Your holistic view that your patient is not merely a diagnosis and is more than just the presenting problem will strengthen both your own commitment and your patient's loyalty to the therapy.
- *Empathy*. Your ability to understand the patient's feelings and point of view, perhaps to express the patient's state of mind when even he or she cannot put it into words, will enhance any therapy approach and promote healing.

These qualities are conveyed not only by your verbal statements but also by nonverbal cues, such as tone of voice and facial expression, and

---

[8]Unconditional positive regard is a concept developed by Carl Rogers (1902–1987) for his client-centered therapy, but it has now become a general therapeutic principle that encompasses the basic acceptance and support of the patient without evaluation and judgment.

by the way you behave toward the person sitting across from you. To strengthen the alliance, follow the biblical injunction, "Do unto others as you would have others do unto you." To the extent that you do not or cannot demonstrate these positive attributes, the alliance will suffer. If you are cool, indifferent, bored, intellectualizing, insensitive, rigid, closed, intolerant, self-interested or take a narrow view of the patient, you will fare poorly in whatever therapeutic modality you seek to employ. Fortunately for the field, few people with these unhelpful attitudes are attracted to this type of career.

Your contribution to the alliance will depend not only on your possession and display of these personal attributes but also on your patient's ability to recognize and accept them. Patients who, as a consequence of earlier deficits, disability, and damage, are unable to appreciate your behavior will have difficulty forming an alliance with you. If distrust, suspicion, delusional ideation, melancholic self-absorption, and other evidences of severe disability are present, your best efforts may only result in a weak and fragile alliance. In those circumstances, the prognosis for successful therapy is guarded.

The Patient's Contribution

The patient's contribution to the alliance includes:

- *Motivation.* The patient must be motivated to change the problem behaviors on which your therapy is focused. Willingness to be "in treatment" is insufficient. (It may arise from social or legal pressures or express dysfunctional family dynamics. Some patients seek out therapy with a misplaced belief in vague, general benefits, like insight, self-actualization, or self-knowledge, that is both unlikely and irrelevant.) Only a genuine interest in and willingness to change the target behaviors will allow your patient to join with you in a useful therapeutic alliance.
- *Honesty.* Psychopaths are untreatable, but all of us have at least a little inherent dishonesty. I think it is fair to say that deceit has been a part of human interaction since the first hominids formed their little bands of hunter-gatherers in the prehistoric past. The degree to which your patient is willing to participate without deception and subterfuge will determine the strength of his or her alliance with you. Over time, your half of the therapeutic alliance—those positive qualities listed above—may overcome the patient's suspicion and distrust, so that the patient becomes more open and revealing as the therapy progresses.

- *Acceptance of the therapeutic rationale.* In the previous chapter,[9] I reviewed the way a therapy relied on a "myth," a coherent explanation of behavior, as one of the basic requirements of therapeutic success. If your patient is unconvinced by your presentation of this rationale, or otherwise unable to accept it, he or she will not join with you in the therapeutic process. Highly intellectualized people with obsessional traits, untrusting individuals with a paranoid stance, and intellectually challenged patients are some of those who can have difficulty with this requirement.
- *Acceptance of the therapeutic process.* Another component of the alliance is your patient's willingness or capacity to participate in the "ritual" elements of the therapy, the techniques and procedures you offer as a path to recovery. While resistance is a constant counterforce to therapeutic progress, one that can be dealt with as part of the therapy, wholesale rejection, skepticism, or serious doubt about the treatment offered will prevent the formation of an effective alliance.
- *Acceptance of the setting as a safe environment.* Privacy and confidentiality are requirements of generic psychotherapy that must be present and accepted for your patient to trust you and unite with you in the therapeutic effort.
- *Respect for the therapist.* Although you are entitled to the social role of healer by virtue of your training and experience, and you have the credentials to back it up, some patients will not accept your bona fides and will as a result hesitate to accept you. Sometimes this reluctance is based on perceived personal differences—gender, race, ethnicity, etc.— and may also yield over time as the patient becomes more comfortable with you.
- *Expectation of a successful outcome.* For some people, the glass is always half empty. The patient who is deeply pessimistic, who is depressed and hopeless, or who lacks the requisite social skills will not form a strong alliance. You may need to address this global problem and bolster the patient's hope and optimism or make a better connection before you can begin to treat the specific difficulties that brought him or her to your office.

A therapeutic alliance is never static or monolithic. The various elements that go into its creation—all of the attitudes and assumptions listed above—will vary in intensity over the course of treatment. Because the patient's perceptions fluctuate, so does the strength of the al-

---

[9]See pages 37–38.

liance. It is usually strong at the beginning, before therapy gets solidly under way. As problems arise in the therapy and the therapist's actions impose stress on the patient, the alliance may recede or even rupture, but once repaired by further therapeutic work, it will become again a potent healing force. It may be strongest as therapy approaches its conclusion. Figure 3–1 illustrates this progression.

Strengthening the Alliance

The therapeutic alliance, by itself, has substantial therapeutic value. Some significant portion of the patient's improvement, perhaps half (although this estimate is only an educated guess), occurs solely as a result of the alliance. Patients may improve after a single consultation or even while on a waiting list, without any apparent therapy taking place. The beneficial effect seen in these apparently nontherapeutic contacts results from the placebo effect and perhaps the nonspecific factors described in the previous chapter and may reflect the hopeful expectation they engender. Another way to think about this effect is that human beings have an intrinsic ability to heal, if conditions allow, and that the therapeutic alliance fosters these healing conditions.

Some would argue that the alliance provides all, or almost all, of the success of any therapy, and that the methodology is merely an epiphenomenon or a vehicle by which the healing effects of the alliance can be delivered. It does not matter, so this argument goes, whether that methodology is exploratory, directive, or experiential. As long as the patient accepts it and participates, therapy will have a positive outcome. This explanation says that all types of therapy are merely different formats for communication between the two participants and that it is the communication itself (as a representation of the alliance) that affects the patient's behavior. I am not persuaded that that argument is valid (or maybe I don't want it to be true), but it is certainly clear that the therapeutic alliance

- Does involve communication between the two participants.
- Is necessary if the therapy used is to change the patient's behavior.

Although the alliance may be necessary for therapeutic improvement, and despite the idea of methodology as an epiphenomenon, it is usually not sufficient by itself. In any case, it is also clear that the alliance

- Has a strong positive effect on the outcome of any therapy.
- Enhances patient cooperation and thus makes possible the successful application of whatever technique the therapist employs.

Given this importance, you must do everything possible to establish, maintain, and strengthen the alliance. Since it is the result of the totality of the patient's perception of you, every detail of your appearance and your environment will have an effect on your psychotherapy relationship. Three important factors that help to create this effect are

- The therapeutic setting.
- Your professional presentation or role.
- Your demeanor.

The Therapeutic Setting

The primary purpose of a psychotherapy office is to provide the safe environment that is a necessary component of the healing paradigm discussed in the last chapter. The location of that safe setting in a professional site can provide an additional benefit if it supports your social standing as a recognized expert. You might be able to provide a successful course of therapy in a coffee shop or walking in the woods.[10] You can certainly be a successful therapist working from an office in your home, as many have. A specialized setting, however, will further enhance your effectiveness. A professional building or at least an area with other health service offices will better establish your community position.

Inside the office, you can do more. Unless the place where you and your patient meet has been provided by someone else—an employer, for example—or is not yours to control (like a shared office), you can construct an environment that facilitates therapeutic progress. Important factors to consider include sound, light, furnishings (especially chairs), overall decor, and the geography of the room.

Perhaps it strikes you that a discussion of the physical attributes of a psychotherapy setting reduces a lofty enterprise to a mundane, even trivial, level. Keep in mind that psychotherapy is a relatively weak treatment, compared with, say, curing pneumonia with a course of antibiotics or surgically removing an inflamed appendix. We cannot coerce patients to change; we can only persuade them to do so. Anything that can contribute to the success of that effort is worthwhile, and a propitious physical setting can make a small but significant contribution.

---

[10]Sándor Ferenczi, a member of Freud's inner circle, tried to psychoanalyze a patient on horseback on their daily ride through a Viennese park.

Sound Control

You must completely soundproof the consulting office to guarantee privacy and confidentiality. Nothing will upset waiting patients more than to overhear a therapy discussion and to then realize that others can hear them. If you cannot control the sound, your patient will not feel safe to engage in the therapy there. Short of hiring a soundproofing engineer, some steps you can take include:

- Build office walls that separate the offices from each other and from the waiting room using partitions with staggered studs and an internal sound barrier (Figure 3–2).
- Identify any openings that let sound pass, not only ventilation ducts but even small gaps. Sound is like water on a leaky roof; it will find a way through.
- For existing walls that bleed sound, add a layer of soundproofing material and another layer of wallboard or, better yet, add a staggered stud layer.
- Use soundproofed doors or, almost equally effective, apply weatherstripping to a solid door.
- Consider double doors with weather stripping—one opening in and the other opening out, which are even more effective.
- Place a white noise machine in the waiting area as an added safeguard. Test the result by playing broadcast or recorded sounds in the office and listening for any sound leakage in the waiting area.

Light

Natural lighting is best during the day, provided the window treatments ensure privacy, and after dark, lighting should approximate the daytime ambience. Avoid a dim shadowy room or one glaringly bright. You want the patient to feel safely illuminated but not under interrogation.

Furnishings

Set up the consulting room for comfort with a professional atmosphere.

- The minimal furniture needed is two chairs, one for you and one for the patient.
- Two "patient chairs" are better, separated by a side table with the traditional box of tissues that says "emotion expected and prepared for."
- A small sofa will also be useful for any larger meeting.

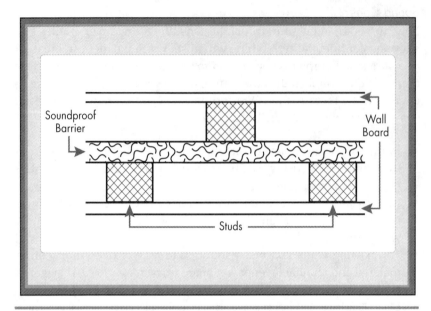

FIGURE 3–2. Soundproofed wall: staggered-stud partition.

Whatever furnishings and decorative items you introduce will communicate to the patient information about your personal and your professional status. With this goal in mind, the furnishings and decor
should be carefully chosen, and the signs of your professional status
should be enhanced. As an example of what *not* to do, I recall a meeting
in one psychoanalyst's office: instead of a couch, he had a double bed with
brass headboard and gold duvet that suggested a seduction more than
a consultation. Your office should not look like your bedroom or your
living room nor should it be a sterile, examining room environment.

Chairs
Your personal chair should be as comfortable and ergonomic as possible. Unlike the patients, you will be sitting there for many hours. Avoid
a big discrepancy, however, between your chair and the patients'. If you
have a sleek, top-of-the-line, ergonomically engineered seat with its
own ottoman, where you lean back with your feet up, but the patients'
chair is a cheaper, standard design where they sit upright with feet on
the floor, the contrast will invite resentment and damage the therapeutic
alliance. Patients will conclude you have a low opinion of them and too
high an opinion of yourself.

Décor

The office should reflect your professional status.

- Hang two or three certificates (but not a whole "wall of fame") and stock a bookcase with reference volumes.
- Avoid pictures of yourself (for example, getting awards or shaking famous hands) and of your family.
- If you include a desk, it should be separate from the seating group, with its own chair. The implication of sitting behind a desk, with the patient across from or beside it, sends the wrong therapy message.
- Remember that anything personal in your office will tell the patient more about you than it may be helpful for them to know. Your choice of paintings, your bric-a-brac, even what kind of pen you use will create an impression, although not necessarily a correct one. Appropriate self-disclosure can be useful, but it should be your choice.

Room Geography

The layout of the room will also exert an influence (Figure 3–3).

- *Distance.* Sit at a comfortable distance from the patient: far enough to easily see the whole person and whatever nonverbal messages are available, but not so far that patients feel they are in the witness chair.

  - ➢ This ideal distance varies among cultures, as you can see when two ethnically diverse people with different comfort zones are standing together in conversation. One person keeps retreating and the other moves forward to close the gap. This awkward dance ends only when the first person has been backed against the wall.
  - ➢ In your office you will "feel" what is the right distance. Keep in mind that at your comfortable distance, the patient may feel too close or too far away and may want to move the chair accordingly.

- *The exit.* Try to set the chairs so that the patient is not between you and the door.

  - ➢ Therapy deals in aroused emotions and sometimes (fortunately, rarely) brings you into contact with people who can become violent. In the unlikely event you need to escape from the room, you do not want the patient blocking you from the door.
  - ➢ Of more usual importance is the need for the patient to leave smoothly at the conclusion of a session. The end of the scheduled

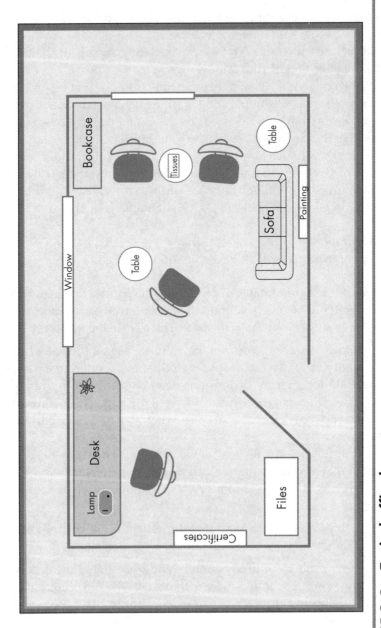

FIGURE 3–3. Typical office layout.

time is an arbitrary stopping point, and the patient will often feel frustrated and unhappy that the session is over. The moment of separation presents a painful loss: the patient will not have further contact with you until the next meeting. These considerations mean that, ideally, the way out should be equidistant from you and the patient, so that on leaving the patient moves away from you toward the door.

In summary, keep in mind that the office will be a source of information for patients: wall color and carpeting, artwork, bookshelf contents, plants, even the presence of a coatrack, along with everything else you "display," will communicate an image of who you are. Think carefully, then, about what your office says about you and whether you are comfortable with that message.

Professional Presentation

You cannot change your age, sex, general physical appearance, height, weight, voice, or mannerisms. You can control your style of dress and general demeanor.

Clothing

How you dress for the office is a strong message to your patients about who you are and what they can expect from you. On the one hand, your choice of wardrobe and grooming must be comfortable for you and represent who you want to be. On the other hand, you should be aware of what message it sends and whether that is the statement you want to make. Consider these two examples:

- Norman Neophyte comes to work wearing a green pullover sweater over a blue oxford dress shirt, open collar, and no tie. He has on gray "Weekday Warrior" slim-fit cotton pants, gray socks, and Nike Lunar Caldra training shoes. His hair is uncombed, and he has a two- or three-day stubble beard.
  - ➤ Norman's clothes would say: "I'm just an ordinary guy, casual and relaxed. I could be your friend."
  - ➤ If we asked him about his choices, he might say. "I like to be comfortable when I work. Besides, formal dress might put people off. I'm more accessible this way."
- Sally Skillful wears an Ann Taylor blue tropical wool suit over a petite-stripe button-down shirt, fastened at the collar, with a strand of pearls and pearl stud earrings. Her shoes are comfortable black flats

over gray silk socks. Sally wears her hair in a short style that falls just below her ears and to her collar in back. Her light makeup uses natural colors.

> ➢ Sally's outfit would declare, "I'm a professional woman with a thoughtful purpose. I'm competent to help you with your problems."
> ➢ Sally herself might say, "I like to be taken seriously. I want people to recognize my professional competence."

We might be tempted to draw some conclusions about how successful each of the two therapists would be in their day-to-day practices, but we cannot tell from simply knowing how they dress. We also need to know what kind of patients they plan to see. How would each of them do if the patient was a rebellious adolescent? A 35-year-old businessman? A middle-aged woman facing a divorce? A retired engineer in his 60s? A better question might be, "Which style of dress gives the therapist more flexibility, the capacity to establish a therapeutic alliance with many patients?"

Of the two presentations, Norman's seems the more limited. Sally's attire seems more flexible. She would be able to quickly and effectively adapt her appearance. For example, she could simply take off her jacket to present a less formal look. Perhaps Norman could more easily interact with younger patients, but he might be at a disadvantage with patients older than he is, who might wonder if he was professional enough to help them. Sally could treat an adolescent or a senior citizen. With the first, she might be viewed as a teacher; with the second, as a contemporary. Norman might hit it off with a patient with multiple facial piercings and full-sleeve tattoos. He might do well with a young computer nerd. It might be more difficult for him to connect with a Type A business person or a depressed government worker, but who knows? Both the informal and formal styles of dress will cause conflict with some patients—you can't please everybody—but Sally's more professional presentation should enable her to deal with a greater range of patients with the least amount of dissonance. She will be able to focus the therapy on more important issues, the central problems the patient brings to therapy, and will spend less time on establishing a strong therapeutic alliance.

Norman's hope that he can be the patient's friend is unrealistic, given the asymmetric relationship discussed earlier, and could arouse conflict between his pretended role as friend and his actual role as therapist. He also might need to think about whether it is more important to be comfortable in the office or to be as effective as he can be. On balance, given the same set of patients and the way they present themselves, Sally might be successful more of the time than Norman.

Demeanor

The therapist's demeanor sets the tone for the session. Again, informality and social niceties contradict the purpose of the therapy, which is a sober and professional effort to help the patient with serious problems. Greeting the patient with a friendly grin and a handshake undermines the effort and invites the patient to mistake the meeting for a social hour or, worse, sends the message that their troubles are of little interest to you. It is rarely necessary to touch the patient—maybe a handshake under special circumstances—and the rare word "never" certainly applies to any flirtatious or sexual behavior.

Critical Therapist Characteristics

Empathy and Narcissism

The most important quality you can bring to your work is *empathy*, the ability to understand and share the feelings of another. The capacity for empathy is an inborn trait that owes its development to the nurturing environment of early postnatal life. Empathy is the reciprocal of narcissistic regard. The narcissistic approach employs self-reference to make sense of another person's behavior. In effect it says, "This is the way I feel, or would feel, about it, so you must feel the same way." To the extent that people share "universal" feelings and reactions—that we all get hungry or experience grief after a loss—the self-referential approach can provide a general sense of what someone else in the same circumstances might feel. Narcissism is useful in normative judgments—how behavior might be viewed in general—but it ignores the specific response of the individual.

Empathy depends on the ability to lower the partition between yourself and another and experience that person's ideas and emotions. A useful analogy is the stimulus barrier. Suppose you are reading this page while birds twitter outside, a TV is playing down the hall, and two people across the room are engaged in a quiet conversation. Your ability to exclude these sounds allows you to keep your attention on this paragraph. Without your stimulus barrier, you might not be able to finish this sentence. You can lower this barrier, however, if you are sitting on a beach, appreciating the sound of the waves, the quality of the sunlight, the warmth of the sun on your skin, even as you look through a magazine. In the same way, a narcissistic barrier excludes the emotional impact of other people and inclines you to focus on your inner thoughts and feelings.

Your narcissistic barrier protects you from the contagion of another person's upset. Medical personnel—physicians, nurses, physician assistants—for example, must use this barrier to maintain enough objective distance to deal effectively with patients in pain, to isolate themselves from the sights, sounds, and smells of disease and from the emotional impact of their patients' disability and approaching death. To be an empathic therapist, however, you must be able to lower this barrier in order to understand a patient on an emotional level. This kind of exposure can take its toll. Being bombarded with raw feelings over the course of several therapy sessions can leave you in need of self-repair at the end of the day. The more sensitive you are to the patient's emotional life, the more successful the therapy will be. At the same time, this sensitivity will create more stress for you than for someone who maintains a better narcissistic barrier to patients. How you regulate these two attributes will determine both how effective you can be as a therapist and how vulnerable you might become to burnout.

Empathy cannot be instilled in someone who lacks the capacity for it, but it can be developed. To maximize your own sensitivity, pay attention not only to what is said but to the associated feelings (the words *and* the music), especially when they are discordant. If the feelings contradict the words or offer a different meaning, focus on the feelings. To improve your receptivity, operate on the patient's wavelength:

- *Pitch your diction at or slightly above the patient's.* Your choice of words and the complexity of your message should mirror the patient. A less educated person may require the occasional four-letter word; with a highly educated patient, an occasional four-syllable word is appropriate. For example, with the first you might say a politician is sneaky; with the second, you might say duplicitous. One patient may respond better to simple declarative sentences and concise ideas; another may respond to subjunctive clauses and more abstract concepts.
- *Maintain eye contact and attention.* Monitor facial expressions, body posture and movements, voice tones, and other nonverbal messages and respond to these when they appear the more important channel of communication.
- *Be sensitive to your empathic facility.* Empathy should help you understand not only the adult in front of you but also the child within. If empathy is putting yourself into another's shoes, learn to put yourself into the little kid shoes in which your patient took those early tentative steps and still puts on at moments of stress or emotional crisis.

Connection

The degree of personal warmth and concern that you show the patient helps the alliance. The distant, blank-faced interviewer, perhaps attempting to evoke the supposedly neutral role of the psychoanalyst, is likely to convey indifference and detachment rather than acceptance and nonintrusive interest.

- Sensitivity and a tolerance for quirks and eccentricities are more helpful than a judgmental or (worse) a mocking attitude.
- The patient should perceive you as flexible and creative, someone who expresses himself or herself with clarity and who demonstrates a capacity for intuition, integrity, and a commitment to the patient's dignity.
- Maintaining the relationship requires respectful address, no humor at the patient's expense, and respect for confidentiality, especially with family members and other interested parties.
- Informed consent and the prior understanding that you will keep no secrets from the patient are important. The therapist is interested *only* in the patient's welfare.

Burnout

All of the above qualities begin to disappear with the development of *burnout*, the emotional, mental, and physical exhaustion brought on by unrelieved and prolonged occupational stress. Burnout results from feeling overwhelmed and unable to meet the constant demands of your work. It corrodes the skills you need to deal with day-to-day problems and responsibilities while it saps your motivation for the job.

The time to combat burnout is before it starts. To do that, build in stress-relieving aspects of your work at the beginning.

- Set limits on your hours and take short, frequent vacations.
- Devote time to outside interests, hobbies, and sports.
- In fee-for-service practice, the temptation is to work longer hours because it generates more income. Instead, decide on a reasonable financial target and set your hours accordingly.
- In salaried positions, know your limits and take on no more responsibility than you think you can handle.
- Select the patients you accept to make sure that the mix does not tilt in favor of those who require more than average intensity. Patients with borderline personality disorder, dissociative identity problems,

high suicidal risk, a tendency to end up in the emergency room—all of these and more can exhaust your store of reserve energy and your tolerance for uncertainty and risk.

- Take advantage of opportunities for peer group associations. Whether as part of a local group of professional friends or at a national conference, the chance to share shoptalk and to network will help to offset the isolation of clinical practice.

Critical Patient Characteristics

The patient's personality and behavior contribute equally to the therapeutic alliance. Some of the key contributions include the following patient attributes:

- *Emotional intelligence.* This term refers to a person's capacity to be aware of, control, and express emotions, and to exercise judgment and empathy in interpersonal relationships. Rigid, intellectualizing patients and those with poor personal boundaries may allow, respectively, too little or too much emotion into the relationship with you.
- *Capacity to participate in the therapeutic process.* This capacity depends on the strength of several mental abilities, among them, abstraction, memory, attention, and concentration. Patients with mania, dementia, or chronic psychosis, for example, may all struggle with these abilities.
- *Ability to trust, without unreasonable dependency needs.* These attributes are often determined early in life. It is very difficult to modify developmental deficits that occurred before the acquisition of language.
- *Maintenance of interpersonal boundaries.* This requirement includes both a recognition of the real relationship and the self-control to inhibit impulses to reconfigure it into a more personal one. Transference distortions may impinge on this condition later in the treatment.
- *Motivation for treatment and motivation for change.* These two attributes are not the same. This difference might be seen with a patient whose substance abuse generates family and social pressures for treatment, but who does not want to give up the addiction.
- *Previous therapy experience.* This factor includes not only whether a successful past experience creates an expectation of accomplishment but also the "training" that earlier therapies may have instilled in the patient. For example, a patient previously treated with cognitive-behavioral therapy may expect more active direction from you than your psychodynamic approach will provide.

Narcissistic Match

I noted that our ancient ancestors lived in tribes that warred over territory and that hated and feared all outsiders. We, their modern descendants, have not evolved past these primitive traits of xenophobia and genocidal war. From the 1620's through the 1920's, to appropriate their land, the "American tribe" slaughtered millions of indigenous men, women, and children, and today, to acquire territory, the "Islamic Extremists' tribes" are killing anyone who differs from their ideology. Many of our contemporary "tribes" are symbolic—perhaps political, like Democrats and Republicans, or class-based, like the 99% and the 1%—or are based on accidental differences like skin tone or country of birth, but the intertribal hatreds are just as strong and can be just as deadly. These same modern "tribal" differences will sometimes separate therapists and patients and will present another barrier to the therapeutic alliance.

Although little can be done about it, a factor that seems to broadly influence the therapeutic alliance is the extent to which the two people share similar personal characteristics. Differences in sex between therapist and patient—male-female or female-male pairs—may hamper it. Of the two, female therapists treating male patients seem more successful than the reverse. The belief that women seem to have a greater capacity for empathy may be posited to explain this difference. A close match of age, race, culture, class, socioeconomic status, and educational level favors a stronger alliance. Our tribal heritage means we are all more comfortable with other people who closely resemble us and are less comfortable with those who are different. This narcissistic choice implies that unless a therapist is treating his or her identical twin, the only perfect match, then any discrepancy will present a barrier to the therapeutic alliance. Fortunately, all of us share a common humanity, and these basic human traits provide a foundation for building an alliance despite the differences. As a result, you can have therapeutic success with patients who are different from you in any of these aspects.

Some of these barriers may be overcome if you are knowledgeable about the areas in which the patient is different and about which the patient may be a source of information. Sometimes, to strengthen the foundation of the alliance in this manner, you must acknowledge the differences and ask the patient to educate you about them. For example, if your patient is of a different nationality or socioeconomic level, you can ask for an explanation of whatever unfamiliar references may emerge. Be respectful, inquisitive, and open-minded, and these barriers can be reduced by a successful collaboration. Patients will often willingly undertake the role of the expert who can enlighten the otherwise all-knowing therapist in an area of ignorance. Although patients' perceptions of their personal environment may not be accurate and may reflect their own biases, the information they provide represents their version of the subject and, therefore, the reality the therapy needs to deal with.

Cybertherapy and the Therapeutic Alliance

After all the attention we have paid to those human attributes of both therapist and patient that enhance and support the therapeutic alliance, it now appears that computer programs that deliver therapy also enjoy this connection to some degree. Apparently, patients who use a digital, nonhuman therapy program develop some of the same trust and respect for it as they do with human therapists. In cybertherapy, it seems that:

- Patients animate the computer the way children name dolls and treat them as real and the way primitive people animated nature with tree spirits and river gods.
- After the object is endowed with human characteristics, the animated entity can become a quasi-being interested in and caring about the user who imagined it into existence.

To understand this phenomenon, we can look to some basic attributes of human nature. When users animate the computer to create a therapeutic alliance with an inanimate program, they rely on an evolved skill that facilitates our existence as social animals. The user feels connected to the program because it is a fantasied human other. To do so, users must ignore two facts:

- They are participating in a complex digital program.
- There is no "person" in it; the program itself has no interest in or concern for them.

This effect can only be enhanced when the program uses a virtual reality interface and a human avatar to mimic the visual representation of a human being. The program

- Has a voice, facial expressions, and simulated interest and concern.
- Lacks negative judgment, sarcasm, scorn, and perceived indifference.
- Seems safer and more accepting than a person.

The computer appears to be an idealized mother:

- It never gets hungry or sleep-deprived.
- Its attention never wanders.
- It is available at all hours, whenever the patient wants it.
- It consistently provides unconditional positive regard.
- Within its limited assignment, it delivers expert help.

Perhaps we can take some comfort in these observations if we realize that we will receive some of the same attention invested in the computer and that this tendency of patients to form an alliance with any available sympathetic source will also help them to form one with us.

Inability to Form an Alliance

Psychotherapy does not work for everybody. It is not a panacea. At times, you must decline to offer therapy when your best judgment is that the patient is unsuitable. The same pathology responsible for their behavioral difficulties—often arising from personality disorders—makes it unlikely or impossible for them to benefit. Trying to treat those who cannot, or will not, participate in a therapeutic alliance is an exercise in futility. The mental health problems of these patients will need treatment by some means other than psychotherapy.

The following, incomplete list of pertinent pathologies is suggested as a guide:

- Neurodevelopmental disorders
  - ➤ Patients with intellectual disability severe enough to impact language and social skills will be incapable of connecting with the therapist.
  - ➤ Some patients with autism spectrum disorder will be unable to form an interpersonal relationship.
- Psychotic disorders
  - ➤ Delusional patients with prominent paranoia will not form a realistic or trusting relationship.
  - ➤ Manic patients or those with severe agitation are too distractible and energized to attend to the therapist.
- Paraphilic disorders
  - ➤ Motivation for treatment is usually external for patients with paraphilic disorders; often they are responding to legal duress.

➤ Experience shows that patients with pedophilia, sadomasochism, and other disorders in this group are, at least at present, impervious to a psychotherapeutic effort.

- Personality disorders
  ➤ We all have some questionable personality traits, even though their severity and number do not add up to a formal diagnosis. Personality traits that fall within one or more of the diagnostic categories, even if not sufficient to meet criteria for a personality disorder diagnosis, will nevertheless impact the success or failure of the psychotherapy. You may be able to recognize an unsuitable patient when confronted with a fully developed disorder. You will find it more difficult when your potential patient displays only some of the problematic characteristics or they are only partially manifested. Patients with

  - Paranoid traits may not trust the therapist.
  - Schizoid traits may form a meaningful relationship with great difficulty.
  - Schizotypal traits may not tolerate a close relationship.
  - Narcissistic traits lack empathy.

- Psychopathic (antisocial) personality
  ➤ One type of patient who is easily mistaken for treatable is the clever psychopath. (The psychopath who is not cunning and adroit is headed for prison or is already there.) These patients may give the appearance of normality, but their history of antisocial behavior shows that they use this façade for deceit and manipulation. Clever, intelligent psychopaths are often astoundingly successful. Think of Bernie Madoff's decades-long Ponzi scheme that only collapsed when exposed by the severe recession of 2008. Absent some unexpected reversal, the Madoffs of the world may avoid the legal consequences of their antisocial behavior and never be caught.[11]

  The clever psychopath will only seek your help when external pressures, often involving legal jeopardy, require him (or, occasionally, her) to look for cover in a psychiatric setting. Sometimes

---

[11]Perhaps not surprisingly, psychopathy is correlated with the highest levels of personal success. Those who study the personality profiles of U.S. Presidents and the Chief Executives of major corporations report that psychopathic traits are more common in these groups than in the general population. Think of Richard Nixon and Bill Clinton, and the top executives of Enron and Countrywide Mortgage.

a psychopath's search for therapy results from successful prosecution when treatment is a requirement of probation or parole, but it may also stem from the anticipation of threat. In any case, these people will only manipulate you, involvement with them will sometimes prove damaging, and you should decline to treat them. If a clever psychopath comes to you for therapy, you might not be able to spot his psychopathy until he gets what he wants and moves on. The only hope of avoiding these unsuitable, and possibly dangerous, patients is to maintain a high index of suspicion in every consultation.

OPERATIONAL PLAN

The third component of the psychotherapy relationship is the interaction of therapist and patient in the operation of the treatment plan. The plan might confine itself to a single methodology or it might use a combination of methods. For example, a plan to use cognitive therapy to treat a depression might need a psychodynamic approach to deal with an intercurrent transference problem. Whichever of the multitude of psychotherapies available is used, whether it is highly structured like a behavioral treatment or loosely constructed like an existential encounter, the two participants must engage in a reciprocal process of communication and constructive influence.

I estimated that the therapeutic alliance usually accounted for half of the therapeutic benefit. The operational plan provides the other half, but the ratio is not always fifty-fifty. Instead, the balance changes, sometimes from one session to the next. The operational plan becomes increasingly important as therapy progresses, fueled by (but also weakening) the therapeutic alliance, and then tapers off as the therapy nears termination. This "ideal" pattern is shown in Figure 3–4. In reality, however, the course of therapy, like that of true love, "ne'er did run smooth."

In practical terms, this duality means you cannot help people by the therapeutic alliance alone, but you can build a successful therapy on the foundation it provides. The more solid the foundation the better the methodology will succeed. Which therapeutic modality to choose and whether to select different methodologies for each therapy goal are discussed in Chapter Six. Once the treatment plan is completed, you must have a therapeutic agreement with the patient. The process of negotiation by which the agreement is reached will depend on the trust, understanding, and hopeful expectation the alliance provides. Once underway, the strength of the alliance will determine the patient's willingness to persevere and the intensity of the inevitable resistance that will develop.

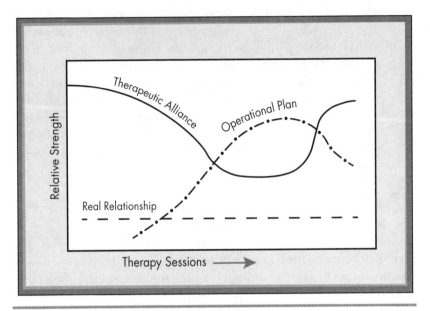

FIGURE 3-4. **Ideal psychotherapy.**

The absence of an operational plan is often misnamed "supportive therapy." Without a plan, you are left with only the therapeutic alliance and perhaps some direct advice. Another way of looking at this third piece of the psychotherapy relationship is that "support" is present in every therapy as a nonspecific underpinning of each particular methodology. Yet another way of thinking about this aspect of treatment is that when you offer only support, you have no operational plan at all. Although support is generally necessary, it is not usually sufficient to bring about the desired therapeutic change.

Final Thoughts

The general relationship between you and your patient is of at least equal importance with the specific methods you use in your treatment. Early in the therapy, in fact, the alliance is the more important factor, and future success will depend on its strength and suitability. Later, at the height of the therapeutic effort, the relationship is less obviously at work, but it, nevertheless, provides the underpinnings for the ongoing treatment. This principle suggests that you should continue to monitor the relationship, be sensitive to any deterioration it may undergo, and repair any breach or rupture that occurs. In effect, you must operate along two parallel tracks: the state of the alliance and the progress of the methodology, and devote equal attention and energy to both.

Key Points

- The psychotherapy relationship is a therapeutic force that accounts for a significant portion of the patient's improvement.

- The three components of psychotherapy are the real relationship, the therapeutic alliance, and the operational plan.

- The real relationship includes a recognition of the extratherapeutic attributes of both parties and the administrative aspects of their collaboration.

- The therapeutic alliance develops from the personal qualities of each participant and is enhanced by cultural expectations and the physical environment.

- The therapeutic alliance has considerable positive influence on the therapy results.

- The failure to form a strong alliance, no matter if the therapist or the patient is responsible, will damage the therapy and diminish the likelihood of a favorable outcome.

- The operational plan, with its agreed-upon therapy goals and methodology, may cause the therapeutic alliance to weaken or even rupture over the course of treatment.

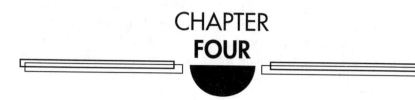

CHAPTER
FOUR

What Is an Initial Evaluation?

"The time has come," the Walrus said,
    "to talk of many things:
Of shoes—and ships—and sealing-wax
Of cabbages—and kings—
And why the sea is boiling hot—
    And whether pigs have wings."

Lewis Carroll

You can observe a lot by watching.

Yogi Berra

Introduction

The first meeting between you and a patient often generates anxiety in both. For you, the source of apprehension includes

- The often skimpy referral information that generates uncertainty about what challenges you will face.
- Concern over the need to establish a good working relationship.

For the patient, the additional worry reflects

- The conflict between hope for assistance and skepticism about your ability to provide it.
- The tensions produced by whatever prejudices, fantasies, and wishes have been building since the referral.

All of these concerns endow the meeting with heightened significance. Whatever the two of you expect is immediately confronted by the

107

reality of your perceptions and the first exchanges that follow. That reality begins to reduce the emotional intensity, and most of the time, you and the patient settle into a productive discussion. Occasionally, however, problems that arise from the first meeting cannot be overcome and the therapy fails.

A Singular Experience

The initial interview is unique. You and the patient meet without prior involvement, an opportunity to make a first impression that may set the tone for the rest of the therapy. Your meeting has a dual purpose:

1. Your therapeutic relationship starts with the first contact, and you must immediately begin to develop and solidify the therapeutic alliance.
2. You must gather the data and make the judgments needed to evaluate the patient for future treatment and then plan a possible course of therapy.

In this chapter, I will discuss the type of evaluation that will allow you to prepare a course of psychotherapy. Whole books have been written about the initial interview, and it is, of course, conducted for other purposes as well, such as

- Forensic examinations.
- Disability evaluations.
- Medication management.
- Consultations for another health professional.

This discussion is limited to interviews conducted for the initiation of a course of psychotherapy. A therapy evaluation is different from a diagnostic interview or one done for a general assessment because its purpose is to assess whether the patient

- Needs treatment.
- Has a problem therapy can help.
- Is someone you want to accept in therapy.

You will also determine

- What diagnosis best fits the patient's presentation.
- What problems require treatment.
- The best treatment approach.

To meet these requirements, you must decide how to budget the available time to

- Make a diagnosis.
- Develop a history.
- Evaluate the patient for treatment.
- Formulate the case.

The initial evaluation has a long agenda, and it may not be possible to accomplish it all in one interview, even if you set aside extra time for this purpose. Pressure from third-party payers will incline you to be as efficient as possible, but sometimes the patient's presentation is simply too complex to wrap everything up in a single session.

The Semistructured Interview

The format for an initial interview should strike a balance between structured questions and an open-ended approach. A fully structured interview—with a set of questions preselected and organized into a list—might be appropriate for a research project. A totally unstructured interview—perhaps with only one request: "Tell me about yourself"—is useful for a correspondingly unstructured treatment, such as classical psychoanalysis. In general, for most psychotherapy you need a format midway between the two, with some open-ended questions to elicit what the patient thinks is important and some structured questions to acquire sufficient information about a significant topic.

The patient's ability to provide information also determines how much you must direct the interview. Some will be able to organize and recount large amounts of relevant information, and others will need your frequent intervention to focus on the important areas or to redirect them to the topic under review. The resulting balance will also determine the "distance" needed for future work; that is, how active or passive you will be in the therapy to follow. Both extremes—a fully structured interview and one completely open-ended—will create more distance, the first because it interposes the questionnaire format between you and the patient, and the second because the less you say, even though you are actively listening, the less you connect with the patient. Both will reduce the intensity of the initial therapeutic alliance, a deficiency that may have negative consequences later on.

Often overlooked in the mix of available sources of information are the records of the patient's prior treatment. Whether treatment was out of state or local, it is always worthwhile to request a report from every identified source of prior care, institutional or private. In each case, you will need the patient's signed release of information agreement and a cover letter giving the dates of service and making the formal request. These outside records are valuable because they

- May include information of which the patient is unaware.
- May uncover facts the patient has forgotten or concealed.
- Furnish an objective assessment of the patient's reliability as a historian.
- Provide an independent evaluation from another professional source.
- Supply important documentation in case of any future legal proceedings.

Instead of a formal request for written records, you can make direct contact with a previous therapist, again with the patient's consent. The advantage, especially if you know the other therapist, is the possibility of a more open, informal, and candid response. The disadvantage is you may not be able to get all the important details, especially if the contact is a brief telephone conversation between two busy professionals. Include both the patient's consent and a summary of the information in the patient's record.

The question will sometimes arise as to how much of this past record should be shared with the patient. Some states provide restrictions on disclosing this information, and others give the patient the legal right to see it, so check on the applicable regulations. As to your own decision, you can tell the patient that you would be willing to reveal any of it, if you are legally permitted to do so, provided that in your judgment it will not impede your current treatment plan.

First Impressions

The initial face-to-face session with the patient is the only meeting you will have without the distortion of a prior encounter. Every subsequent occasion will be influenced by your past experience, the impact of earlier transactions, and the accumulated emotions of your work together. Sometimes the effect of this initial contact will only be apparent at a later point. For example, when a female patient hesitated at the doorway to the office before her first session, I spontaneously ushered her in with a half bow and a sweeping motion of my arm, a courtly gesture that elicited a giggle. Only later did I learn that I had provoked an erotic transference in which she fantasized about me as "Prince Charming."

Your first decision is what to call the patient and how you want the patient to refer to you. The form of address will influence the kind of relationship you will have because it denotes both social status and relative position. Because your choice will be an important factor, it is worth thinking about your options and what they will mean. In most two-person conversations, it is rarely necessary to use the other person's name: you both know who you are talking to. The initial greeting may be one of the few times the use of names will come up, giving it perhaps an additional importance.

Since you are likely to be the first to speak, you can set the tone by how you introduce yourself: first name? both names? title? Consider these options and their possible implications:

- Hi, I'm Jane. (You pretend that you and the patient are social equals and that you are not, in fact, a professional. Remember: psychotherapy is not friendship.)
- Hello, I'm Jane Doe. (Your more formal introduction assumes the patient knows your professional status, but you choose not to emphasize it.)
- Hello, I'm Dr. Jane Doe. (You overtly acknowledge the professional relationship, but you include your first name to soften the formality.)
- Hello, I'm Dr. Doe. (You strongly emphasize your professional status.)
- Hello. Please come into the office. (You assume the patient knows who you are and avoid the whole question of names, at least for the moment.)

The next decision is how you will address the patient. Children, adolescents, and even some young adults expect to be called by their first name. With older adults, you can, and should, use the Mr., Mrs., or Ms. forms of address but probably not the last name alone, thus "Mr. Smith" but not simply "Smith." A title and last name is preferable because it

- Establishes a professional distance.
- Acknowledges the asymmetry of the relationship.
- Enhances your therapeutic influence.
- Is more respectful of the patient.
- Avoids the phony assumption that you are just friends.

If an adult patient uses your title and last name and you reply with her or his first name, you

- Show disrespect, as if you are speaking to an inferior.
- Create an expectation of dependency, as though the patient was a child.
- Invite more informality than is generally useful.
- Diminish your status as a professional.

Occasionally, a patient will request that you use his or her first name. The meaning of this request is worth thinking about or even exploring as a therapy issue. Does the patient consider themselves childlike, an inferior to you? Is it a request for a more personal (less professional) relationship? You may need to explain why you prefer the more formal terms, recognizing that your explanation may be perceived as a rejection.

Information Gathering

An important function of the first session is to gather information about the patient. And, of course, the patient is also accumulating information about you. Both of you, however, may already have some knowledge of the other. You have acquired some ideas from the referral source prior to the initial appointment. Your patient will arrive with a set of expectations and biases, perhaps based on prior treatment, cultural stereotyping, or personal ideas about therapists in general. It is likely that your patient has tried to find out more about you, perhaps including some degree of online research both about psychotherapy in general (especially the type you are known to provide) and about you in particular.

If you have information from an outside source—whether from another professional or from a family member or friend—it may be helpful to begin by telling the patient what you know. You can simply say, "I heard from Dr. Smith (or your mother, sister, friend, etc.) that you're having a problem with (fill in the blank). Let me tell you what they said, and then you can give me your own ideas." This opening helps you to establish trust: you will not keep secrets, and your patient has the last word. In addition, it will "break the ice" and put the focus on the patient's reason for coming.

If you do not have enough referral information to justify this type of start, then the best opening is "What can I do for you?" or some variation of it. Such a statement establishes from your first words that you

- Want to help the patient with something specific.
- Are interested in what the patient considers important.
- Expect the patient to collaborate in defining the task.

You will strengthen this idea of therapy as a collaboration later on, after you have a treatment plan and can invite the patient to accept it.

The initial interview should establish a diagnosis, even though it may not be very useful in developing a treatment plan. Psychiatric diagnoses are somewhat arbitrary descriptions of observed behavior and subjective mental states. Their uniform specifications are useful to establish a common framework for research or epidemiological studies. Most have no (as yet) known foundation in physiology. At this stage in our knowledge of the brain, the scientific method is not the basis for diagnostic accuracy. Unlike modern medicine, we do not know enough to provide an etiology for most of the diagnostic categories. Psychiatric diagnoses are decided by committees assembled for each new version of the diagnostic manual. Sometimes the committees are influenced by political and social considerations. In 1974, for example, after several years of protests by gay activists, the American Psychiatric Association decided by a vote of the trustees (13–0, with 2 abstentions) and then by a vote of the membership (5,854 out of 10,555 votes or about 55%) that homosexuality was not a mental illness. Note that this "majority" was only 32% of the total membership of 17,905. Nevertheless, the minority got it right, and same-sex preference was no longer the basis of a disorder.

In spite of its limitations, you will need a diagnosis for

- Completing the clinical record.
- Communicating with other interested parties, including other caregivers and, at times, courts and other social institutions.
- Submitting claims for payment to third parties.

The diagnosis will not determine the best treatment. A particular therapy method can usually be applied to many different diagnostic categories. Knowing the diagnosis does not help to predict the outcome of a course of treatment.

Not much of the initial interview's valuable time should be required to make the diagnosis. Experienced practitioners usually arrive at a diagnosis very soon after beginning the interview, often within the first three or four minutes. Not only do the patient's first words help in reaching this conclusion, but together with nonverbal information—posture, body language, facial expression—all create an early impression that may be modified by later observations but is often correct. What this early decision means is that you can spend the great majority of the interview on arriving at a formulation and narrowing your ideas about the treatment needed.

And, by the way, avoid the temptation to objectify patients by reducing them to their diagnosis:

- Not "an alcoholic," but a teenager with alcohol dependence
- Not "a schizophrenic," but a man with schizophrenia
- Not "a borderline," but a woman with borderline problems

To think of patients as merely a diagnosis distances you from their unique, individual problems and invites stereotyped condemnation: alcoholics are drunks, schizophrenics are crazies, borderlines are patients from hell. Treatment that starts with the dehumanization of the patient is already at a disadvantage.

WHAT TO LOOK FOR

In response to your opening question ("What can I do for you?"), most patients will respond with a frank recital of what is troubling them. You can help this recitation along with appropriate comments and questions, but, in general, you should allow patients to get the story out as fully as they wish. Try not to impede the effort the patient makes to inform you and to explain the whole situation by interrupting with questions that can wait or jumping in with unnecessary comments and ideas. At times, this opening explanation includes a good deal of emotion, a type of catharsis, because the patient may not have previously revealed these problems to anyone else. Your attitude of nonjudgmental interest and impartial concern will help to facilitate the release of these feelings.

What patients choose to tell you and how they present their story will usually reflect what is of the greatest importance to them, regardless of what you might want to hear. In the words of Holden Caulfield,

> If you really want to hear about it, the first thing you'll probably want to know is where I was born, and what my lousy childhood was like, and how my parents were occupied and all before they had me, and all that David Copperfield kind of crap, but I don't feel like going into it, if you want to know the truth. In the first place, that stuff bores me...Besides, I'm not going to tell you my whole goddam autobiography or anything. I'll just tell you about this madman stuff that happened to me around last Christmas just before I got pretty run-down and had to come out here and take it easy.[1]

---

[1]Salinger, JD: *The Catcher in the Rye.* Little, Brown and Company, 1951.

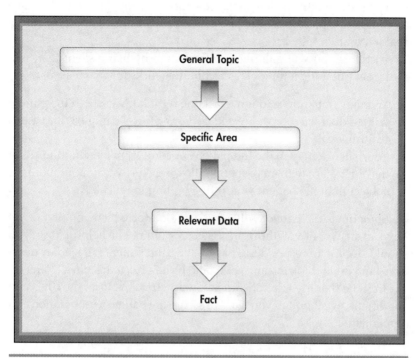

FIGURE 4–1. Progressive line of inquiry.

Once the patient has described his or her presenting difficulties, you can become more active in your investigation. Your questions should be asked in the service of your effort to formulate the patient's problems in a way that allows you to decide on a treatment approach. To that end, ask enough questions about a topic to fully comprehend both its present effects and its past sources, or in other words, its antecedents and consequences. Do not settle for an incomplete first explanation or an inadequate initial assertion. Instead, dissect and challenge each statement until you conclude you have a clear understanding of it. This technique requires that you question the first answer, then the next answer, and so on until the subject is fully covered. Each line of inquiry should progress from the general to the particular (Figure 4–1). It is better to understand a single topic completely than it is to have a shallow grasp of many topics. Granted, you will cover less ground with this approach than you would with a standard, medical model history.[2] You do not need to know everything about the patient in this first meeting, but you do need to have as complete a picture as possible of the present illness and everything that led up to it.

At times you will gain more information by being silent than you will from pursuing a topic. This technique works for two reasons:

1. You may not know enough to ask the right question, and the patient will be distracted or redirected by your off-topic inquiry into a less fruitful area.
2. Your silence may make the patient uncomfortable enough to fill in the quiet space with more speech, allowing you to hear more about the subject than the patient was at first willing to reveal.

Sometimes the patient will ask a question for which you do not yet have an answer or you think an answer would not be helpful. If so, you should decline to respond, perhaps telling the patient, "It's a fair question, but I don't think my answer would be helpful at this time." Remember that the therapy relationship is asymmetrical: you set the rules and conditions, even though you want to secure the patient's cooperation and agreement.

When you do pursue a general issue, take a branching inquiry: follow one line of investigation to its end while you take note of other possibilities and then return to the original topic and begin a new search for relevant material (Figure 4–2).

In addition to the verbal account of what the patient wants you to help with, pay attention to other sources of information (Table 4–1):

- *Nonverbal behavior.* Amplifying or modifying the patient's words will be a variety of other behavioral cues:
  - ➤ *Posture.* Is the seated position
    - Closed, with arms across the chest and legs crossed?
    - Open, with arms and legs apart?
    - Dominant, with body taking up as much space as possible?
    - Submissive, with body closed and leaning forward?
  - ➤ *Movement.* Does the patient
    - Fidget? Twiddle a ring? Rub the hands together? Touch the face?

---

[2]The medical model history covers present illness, past history, past psychiatric history, family history, medical history, mental status, and diagnostic impressions.

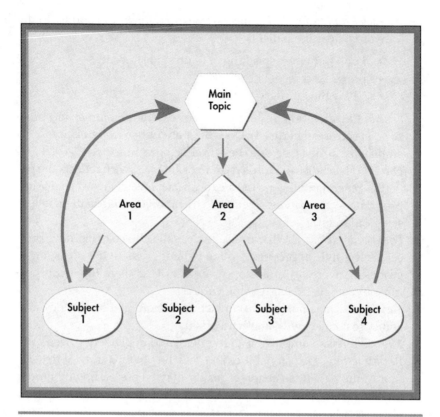

FIGURE 4–2. Branching inquiry.

- Seem immobile? Wince in pain?
- Mirror your position or movements? (This behavior is a positive sign that indicates the patient feels in better rapport or is more engaged with you. Resist the temptation, however, to emulate salespeople, politicians, and other self-interested persuaders who consciously mirror the other person in an attempt to simulate rapport and further their own agendas. This type of manipulation is sure to have unwelcome consequences when the patient realizes what you are doing.)
- Gesticulate to emphasize the spoken message?
- Nose wipe? (Running the fingers under the nose is an unconscious gesture denoting disapproval or negative feelings about the subject of the patient's words.)
- Hunch the shoulders? Flex the ankle? (Tension about a subject is reflected in ankle flexion that raises the foot, either momentarily or for a sustained time.)

> ➤ *Facial expression*, including microexpressions:[3] In contrast to the words, does the patient

- Look sad when speaking of neutral past events?
- Frown and seem angry?
- Chew the lips nervously?

- *Speech.* Pay attention to the tone of voice, strain, volume, and pressure. Is sarcasm overused? Does the patient use irony or humor to emphasize or distance or to be self-effacing?
- *Diction.* The choice of words used in ordinary speech reflects the patient's general intelligence and educational level. Is word choice appropriate to the patient's age and educational level? Is there use of slang or jargon?
- *Dress and grooming.* What message does the choice of clothing project? Is the style appropriate to the patient's age, to the occasion? Is grooming overly careful, sloppy, unkempt? Is there too much perfume or cologne? Is body odor present?
- *Social skills.* Take note of eye contact, conversational proficiency, and ability to connect with another person.
- *Maturity.* Assess impulsivity, judgment, and dependency needs.
- *Reality testing.* Delusional ideation may be obvious but, more commonly, the patient's version of reality may be misleading or simply mistaken. The patient's interpretation of events or assessment of other people can be, and often is, biased or emotionally distorted. You hear only the patient's perspective and other viewpoints may differ. Be alert to attempts at splitting,[4] with the therapist or with significant others. If the only information source is the patient (as it almost always will be in individual therapy), you should maintain a neutral stance and realize that the person or situation described by the patient—even with no conscious attempt at distortion or bias—may, nevertheless, differ from the reality of either. Resist the temptation to condemn, criticize, or praise and do not make decisions based on these reports.

---

[3]*Microexpressions* are brief changes in expression that can indicate underlying emotions.

[4]In *splitting* (black and white thinking, all-or-nothing thinking), the patient sees only one side, either the positive or the negative attributes, of another and does not perceive the mixed qualities of the whole person. The other person is either a saint or the devil. It can be used to promote discord between two people when one is given only a negative description of the other ("Let's you and him fight").

TABLE 4–1. Sources of clinical information

Direct	*Written:* referral, old records *Verbal:* referral, history
Indirect	*Nonverbal:* posture, movement, expression, speech, diction, dress and grooming, social skills, maturity, judgment, mental status, reality testing

A formal mental status examination is often not necessary because the information is already present in the history. The patient's ability to recount distant and recent events will demonstrate memory.[5] Orientation, judgment, and cognitive skills are usually obvious from your observation of the patient. If organic deficits are in question, however, asking a few of the relevant mental status questions may be a worthwhile expenditure of a few minutes of interview time.

Every evaluation should also address questions of safety. Is the patient a danger to himself or herself or to others? Does the patient have suicidal ideas? Is there a plan? Is the patient in a high-risk group, such as those with alcohol, bipolar, or physical problems; the elderly; those with a prior history of suicide attempts; and the like? You may be hesitant to raise these questions "out of the blue," but unless you are certain that the patient is not at risk, they must, at least briefly, be asked.

THE SUITABILITY CONTINUUM

Finally, you should determine where the patient falls within the range of psychological capacity (Figure 4–3). At one extreme, the high-function end, the patient will

- Be of above-average intelligence.
- Show adequate ability to deal with abstract concepts.
- Have good social and verbal skills.
- Be able to tolerate anxiety.

These patients will do well in most therapies, but they are especially suited for introspective and insight-oriented methodologies. At the other extreme, the low-function end, the patient will

---

[5]Keep in mind, however, that memory—anyone's memory—is fallible, malleable, and unreliable. Recollections that seem carved in granite may be, and often are, subjective collections or selective fragments or even total fabrications.

- Be intellectually challenged.
- Be concrete in thinking.
- Have restricted verbal and social skills.
- Have low tolerance for anxiety.

These patients will have a limited ability to benefit from most therapies; they will be best served by case management and directive methodologies.

Most patients' psychological capacity will fall somewhere in the middle of these two extremes. Where you think their capabilities lie will help determine what methodological approach you can offer them and how ambitious or how limited the goals of the therapy should be. To some extent, where the patient falls on this continuum will also determine the strength of the therapeutic alliance, with those patients in the middle forming perhaps the stronger bonds with the therapist.

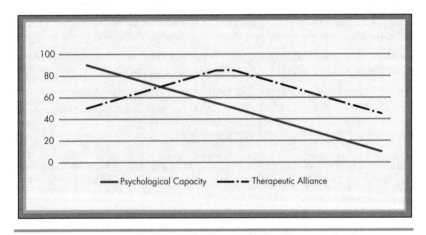

FIGURE 4–3. Continuum of psychological capacity.
Psychological capacity=intelligence, abstraction, social and verbal skills, and tolerance for anxiety.

In assessing this capability, you can be guided by historical information, such as what type and how much education the patient has had, and by observations, such as the kind of vocabulary the patient uses and the ability to grasp whatever concepts you put forward. Mental status questions that test abstracting ability, such as recognizing similarities and differences, might be necessary if other sources of information are not definitive. Although rarely needed, formal psychological testing may be useful too.

Three Key Questions

In addition to the historical facts and the general problem list that the patient will provide, either spontaneously or in answer to your inquiries, the initial interview should provide an answer to the following three questions.

QUESTION 1: WHY DID THE PATIENT COME *HERE?*

It is always useful to know who referred the patient to you. That person can be a source of helpful background information, provided you have the patient's consent to ask for it. How patients found you may also reveal something about their level of trust, their willingness to reveal their problems to another person, and who they felt safe enough to discuss it with. Someone who got your name from an online search may be more uncomfortable with asking for help than a person who can open up at least enough to get a referral from a friend.

This question addresses a subject larger than merely identifying the source of your referral, however valuable that information may be. It arises from the observation that a relatively small number of people with diagnosable mental health or addiction problems seek out an actual mental health care practitioner.

- Many—perhaps three out of four people—do not look for treatment at all. They manage to live with their disability.
- Others consult their primary care provider or other nonpsychiatric physicians. Intense and widespread aggressive marketing by pharmaceutical companies, in combination with the relative scarcity of mental health resources, prompts those with prescriptive authority to give their patients psychiatric medications without consultation with or referral to anyone in the mental health community. The choice of medication over psychotherapy can prevent a patient from getting the best treatment.
- Some look for help from peer groups, such as the various 12-step programs; for example, Alcoholics Anonymous, Gamblers Anonymous, and the like. These programs can be effective, but they deliberately do not include professionals or psychotherapy.
- Non–mental health practitioners, such as life coaches, pastoral counselors, or rehabilitation counselors, offer other services, valuable in their own right, but their assistance is not psychotherapy and does not seek the same outcomes as psychotherapy.

These alternative sources of care avoid one of the main impediments to mental health treatment, the social stigma that persists in spite of all the normalizing efforts to dispel it. They may also cost less and thus attract those with limited means. Whatever factors determine the choice of a psychotherapist instead of other services—educational, social, economic, or theoretical—tell us that the patients who come to our offices are a small, self-selected minority of the large pool of people who could benefit from our help. Why these patients make that choice and what it means to them to have done so are factors whose significance is available in the answer to this first question. That information will help us understand what patients think of themselves and what they expect from us.

QUESTION 2: WHY DID THE PATIENT COME *NOW?*

Many mental health problems are of long standing. Their history may go back years or even decades. At some point in time, the patient decides or recognizes that he or she can no longer carry on the struggle alone. Almost always, you and the patient can identify a precipitating event that immediately preceded the decision to get help. This knowledge is, of course, an important element of the history. It begins the period that we identify as the present illness, even though its antecedents may lie far back in the past. It will often highlight the particular problems that will be the focus of your treatment plan. The information will tell you more, however, than simply what precipitated the referral.

Everyone has a certain ability to cope with stressful life circumstances. As long as the level of stress is manageable and the individual's coping skills are up to the task of containing it, people will be able to function, even if in some discomfort. If they are at the upper limit of these skills, the precipitant may be something trivial, the proverbial straw that supposedly maims the camel. Knowing the precipitant, then, will tell you how close to breaking the patient was beforehand. The intensity of the precipitant will also be informative. A major stress (not a straw but a whole bale of hay) means that your patient was well compensated but overwhelmed simply by the magnitude of the event. An example of the straw might be losing a cell phone. An example of the hay bale might be losing a job. In either case, you will have learned an important measure of your patient's general level of function.

Finally, it may be apparent that the breaking point in your patient's ability to cope resulted from the persistence of stress rather than its intensity. Here the relevant analogy is dripping water wearing away the stone. A manageable stress will, nevertheless, over time erode your patient's ability to withstand it. In these cases, rather than an internal impact, the precipitant may be a change in the environment. For example, a woman may have been able to put up with a nagging, overbearing husband for years, until her mother, an important source of emotional support, suddenly dies, and she walks out on him.

QUESTION 3: WHAT DOES THE PATIENT *WANT?*

The more you can learn about the patient, the better, but time is limited, and you will need to direct your efforts at the most important and significant information. To do that, you must know why the patient has come to you—not just the "chief complaint" but the expectations, wishes, and potential requests. You can focus on this larger picture by your opening inquiry. The question "What can I do for you?" or some variation of it, is a direct query to the patient to specify what he or she wants from the therapy.

The reply to this seemingly obvious question is easy to overlook, yet it is the most important of the three. If you do not determine the patient's principal reason for consulting you, you can hardly be in a position to provide the right help. If you cannot meet the request, knowing what it is at least allows you to suggest an alternative and a better focus of the therapy.

You should attempt to understand the answer to this question as clearly and concretely as possible. Vague and abstract wishes, such as "happiness," "feeling better," "no longer nervous or depressed," are not useful in understanding what is needed or in designing a treatment program to help. Rather, you should pursue what would need to change for the patient to be happier, what is the basis for not feeling better, what makes the patient nervous, what does this patient mean by depressed. Even the answers to those inquiries will often need further exploration before their real meaning is clear.

What your patient wants includes a wide variety of requests, more than simply relief from whatever problems the patient offers as the chief complaint. It is sometimes useful to think of this single identified problem as an "admission ticket." It gets the patient in the door and justifies imposing on your time and professional services. The patient may have other difficulties, however, that either are poorly understood or are felt to be less worthy reasons for seeking help. These tacit requests may include unexpected things the patient wants, such as:

- *Administrative help.* The patient may want assistance with an application for benefits, such as disability payments, or with admission to a desired program, for example, an experimental treatment trial. Instead of therapy, the patient wants you to facilitate the paperwork.

- *Clarification.* The patient may hope to better understand the results of an online test or looks to contradict the opinion of the referring provider, thinking that this authority has determined he or she is "crazy" or that his or her physical complaints are "all in my head." In that case, you are being asked to refute another expert's opinion and to conclude the patient does *not* need therapy.
- *Advice.* A patient without a social support system or the ear of a good friend may hope the therapist supplies guidance for a decision or life choice outside the psychological sphere, for instance, a job change. You are in an unwitting audition for the role of a buddy or an advisor, not a therapist.
- *Psychodynamic insight.* This aspiration is sometimes pursued in a quest for self-knowledge, as reflected in Socrates' assertion that "the unexamined life is not worth living," but the patient has no interest in behavioral change, the only measure of therapeutic success. The patient wants you to be an educator or a fellow philosopher, not a therapist.
- *Ventilation.* The patient may want a sympathetic listener, perhaps for grievances that occurred in some personal or employment relationship. The patient has located the problem in other people and thinks no personal changes are needed and therefore no therapy is necessary. This situation is often misinterpreted as a request for "support" or a "sounding board," neither of which would be therapy.
- *Control.* The patient may want to direct the therapy, either to avoid a difficult area or to limit the therapeutic work. Any therapeutic effort would revolve around this power struggle.
- *Rescue.* The patient may feel trapped in a circumstance from which he or she hopes you will offer deliverance; for instance, a bad marriage. You would be the "authority" that could justify a covert decision the patient has already made.
- *Confession.* The patient may seek absolution through sharing with you something considered shameful or culpable. Your nonjudgmental stance as a therapist would be misinterpreted as that of a religious confessor or a favorable judge.
- *Nothing.* The patient was referred through mistake or misunderstanding or was coerced by others in authority. Unless you recognize it, this mismatch between what the patient wants and what you hope to offer would doom the therapy.

These unstated, and perhaps unconscious, requests may be addressed in the planned therapy, although perhaps not the way the patient hopes, but they must first be uncovered. At times, they remain hidden until the therapy is under way and require, first, that they be dealt with and, then, that the treatment plan be revised.

Sometimes the patient is clear about the goals of the therapy, but the therapist understands that they are not possible. For example, a man may want his wife to be more interested in sex or to be more nurturing, goals that cannot be achieved with the wife absent from the therapy. This recognition can then lead to a productive discussion that modifies the objectives to something more obtainable that the patient can accept instead. In this example, the patient could work on his interpersonal skills or his communication difficulties that might, in turn, improve his marital relationship. Still, what the patient wants may be both overt and reasonable. A successful therapy requires collaboration between you and the patient so that the initial treatment plan includes not just what you think should be treated but also what the patient wants help with as well. Determining the answer to this third question provides the basis for that collaboration.

Hypotheses

DESCRIPTION AND PURPOSE

Hypotheses are testable ideas. As you listen to patients' stories and observe their demeanor in the interview, you can begin to form ideas about what kinds of problems they have and how these problems came about. To both listen and to think about what you hear (and to conduct therapy in general), you must operate on two levels at once:

- The outward level is your behavioral interaction with the patient, the part that responds to what the patient says, both verbally and nonverbally, and in general is your "public face" in the interview.
- The inward level is your ongoing evaluation of what is being said. This inner level of scrutiny is usually called the "observing ego."

We all do this to some extent in any social situation as we try to navigate the requirements of the encounter, the management of our own feelings, and the responses we will allow ourselves to make. It is a mark of maturity to regulate and control our impulses to reply to another person or to interact in a group until we have decided how we can and should respond and the manner in which we will do it. As you confront a patient, however, the exercise of this function, the continuous and deliberate use of the observing ego, is a necessary tool of the trade. Without its constant application to observe and monitor both the patient and your selected interventions, you are not conducting the therapy; you are merely having a conversation.

During the initial evaluation (and throughout the therapy), you utilize your observing ego to—silently and internally—review ideas and construct explanations that will clarify the why and how of the patient's presentation. Your goal in this first meeting is to come up with a reasonable formulation of the patient's situation. It may not be the formulation you decide on later, because as you learn more about the patient, the new facts and observations will inevitably modify or even replace these first efforts. How a formulation is constructed and what use is made of it are subjects for later chapters, but the initial evaluation provides the first opportunity to begin this task.

Each hypothesis, then, should be a provisional statement that pulls together some parts of the data available and assigns them meaning. It may be

- Merely a tentative conclusion. For example, hearing an account of several unsuccessful dating relationships, you might infer that a young man has difficulty separating his ideal of a mate from the actual women he asks out. This observation tells you nothing yet about why he applies this standard or how he developed it, but it presents a framework for further inquiry.
- An initial explanation. For example, at a later point in the interview, you may wonder if the young man's idealized standard developed as a replacement fantasy for his mother, who died when he was five.
- A complex interpretation. For example, if you take a psychodynamic approach, you may conclude that his yearning for an ideal partner represents an unresolved oedipal conflict, the resolution of which was blocked by his mother's death.
- The basis for an effort to gather additional relevant information that will support or amend it. For example, you might then ask this patient about his relationship with his father and see if it fits with your oedipal interpretation.

TESTING HYPOTHESES

The initial interview is rarely the place for therapeutic interventions:

- You have not agreed to treat the patient.
- The patient has not agreed to be treated by whatever methodology you have in mind.

- You do not know what treatment approach will be best.
- Lacking a formulation, you may not fully understand what problems should be treated.
- A random intervention might sidetrack the central reason for the consultation: to acquire as much information as you need to understand the patient's problems.

In Chapter Six, I will review how this "bottom-up" approach (starting to treat before you have a plan of treatment) will torpedo your therapy.

The exception to this stricture is an intervention that either tests one of your hypotheses or tries out your intended therapeutic approach to see how the patient will do with it. You can attempt an interpretation or other intervention or try out one of the techniques you hope to use later. How the patient responds may provide additional history or give you a better idea of how suitable the patient is for the treatment you have in mind. Because these interventions are efforts to assess, rather than attempts to bring about therapeutic change, they should be limited endeavors that are not allowed to sidetrack the evaluation. In other words, you are not trying to help the patient; rather, you are trying to determine the validity of an idea or an approach. If successful, you will use it later in the ongoing treatment effort that results.

Completing the Assessment

Near the end of the initial interview, you should transition from the fact-gathering effort into the portion of the interview when you construct and propose a treatment plan. To check whether you have overlooked anything, and as a final inquiry, you can ask the patient at this point, "Is there anything else I should know? Anything I didn't ask about?" If not, you can move on, first, to the decision to treat and, then, if affirmative, to the formulation and the proposed treatment plan.

TO TREAT OR NOT TO TREAT?

So far, you have merely gathered information. Although the patient expects that this effort is a prologue to getting your help, you still need to make a judgment as to whether or not to offer psychotherapy (Table 4–2). This decision rests on a number of factors.

Is the Patient in Crisis?

A psychological crisis is a state of helplessness brought about when a patient is unable to use effective problem-solving or coping skills. Crisis intervention is a short-term process designed to lower the intensity of

TABLE 4–2. Decision to treat

Question	Example
Patient in crisis?	Acutely suicidal
Duty to warn?	Threat to a specific person
Practical?	Available time and money
Motivated?	Referral forced by external pressure
Treatable?	Severe impulse disorder
Insurmountable challenge	Therapist's lack of specific skill
	Too difficult a case
	Strong negative feelings
	Ethical or moral differences

the situation and to restore the patient to a more stable condition. You must decide if you can manage a patient in crisis on an outpatient basis. For example, a suicidal patient may need to be seen every day. A manic patient may not show up for an office visit. If a patient is not suitable for office-based treatment, then you can arrange a referral to the appropriate inpatient program.

An existential crisis is a set of circumstances that threatens the patient's stability or even survival. You may not be the right person to help. For example, a woman who loses her job, becomes homeless as a result, and has no social support system, no family or friends, will not be able to benefit from psychotherapy until she receives help dealing with these catastrophic events. She would, at the least, require active intervention through case management—she needs food, shelter, and other necessities—before she can deal with any psychological problems.

Is There a Duty to Warn?

Most states have enacted statutes about the obligation to protect anyone threatened with immediate and actual physical harm by a patient under your care. The requirement can be mandatory or simply permissive (shielding you from the consequences of your breach of confidentiality). Check your state's requirements. In the event that you carry out this duty, it is unlikely (but not impossible) that you can go forward with an offer of therapy after you have made your report and brought the patient to the attention of the appropriate authorities.

Is Treatment Practical?

You may find that the patient does not have the time and money necessary for the therapy you feel is needed. You may have to arrange a referral that will take these factors into account. For example, if you are consulted by a college student who will spend some of the year in another state, you may only be able to offer crisis intervention or brief therapy, and you may need to coordinate with another therapist in his home town. Or, if it turns out a patient's insurance restricts the amount of care you feel is required, you may be forced to modify your recommendation from what would be best to what can be managed under the restriction.

Does the Patient Want Treatment?

Sometimes prospective patients will conceal or obscure the real reason they have consulted you. For example, instead of therapy they want your support for getting disability from an employer or the government, or they may seek your expert testimony in a legal claim. While you still might accommodate them (provided they finally reveal their true purpose), if they do not want therapy, or even need it, you should not undertake it. The effort will only be a smoke screen and will almost certainly fail.

Does the Patient Want You?

A patient might want a therapist with skills or personal qualities that you do not have. For example, an addicted patient may want substance abuse counseling or an evangelical Christian may want a Christian therapist. If you do not offer addiction services or you are not an evangelical Christian, these patients can be referred elsewhere.

Is the Patient Motivated?

Successful therapy requires both motivation for treatment and motivation for change. External pressures—for example, by family or the courts—may create motivation for treatment, usually as a way to deal with these pressures or to escape the consequences of past behavior. Treatment may be a way to meet a family ultimatum or a condition of probation. Without a concomitant motivation for change, without an internal motivation, a course of treatment will not likely result in a positive change in the patient's behavior. The therapist in these situations only serves as "cover."

Is There a Treatable Condition?

For some patients, even though their behavior may fall within the defined boundaries of mental illness, no effective treatment is available.

Pedophilia, as one instance, will not change in any fundamental way through any current mental health intervention.

Do You Want to Treat This Patient?

- Do you have the skills and the experience to deal with the problems the patient presents? Perhaps this patient would do well in group therapy or needs specialized treatment for anorexia, and you do not run groups or offer therapy for eating disorders.
- Do you have too many difficult patients like this one already? How many stormy, unstable patients with borderline problems can you handle? How many acutely suicidal?
- Do you like the patient? Some patients simply turn you off from the first moment. For example, if the patient is a trial attorney and you hate lawyers, you will not be a good match for a member of the plaintiffs' bar. Whatever this quirk of yours may be, since it arises so immediately, it is unlikely that you will be able to put aside your feelings and help the patient.
- Do you respect the patient? Perhaps you have a strong philosophical or ethical difference; for example, if your position on the abortion debate conflicts with the patient's activism. These disagreements can undermine the therapeutic alliance to the point that it cannot support a successful therapy.

Until you formally accept the patient for treatment, you do not have a legal obligation to treat. You are lawfully entitled to decline to treat someone. It is important to recognize that you will not do well with some patients, and it is in their interest as well as yours not to take them on. If you do not want to treat the patient, for whatever reason, now is the time to say so, in a consultative framework rather than in a therapy context. It is always difficult to turn a patient away, but if you have to, it is best to handle the rejection in as neutral a fashion as possible. Consider such statements as:

- I don't think I can take on someone who needs as much time/attention as you do. I'll help you find someone who can.
- I don't have a current opening in my schedule, but I believe you need someone now. Let me refer you.
- I think you would benefit from [e.g., group therapy, family therapy], but I don't use that approach. Let me see if I can recommend an alternative.

- I must tell you that I have such strong feelings about [trial lawyers, abortion activists, or whatever] that I would be the wrong person to help you with your problems. I can refer you to someone for whom it would not be a problem.

You can make a specific referral if you know someone who might be a better option, or you can supply the patient with two or three names, or you might suggest a specialized institutional program, such as those for eating disorders or substance abuse.

If you want to treat the patient—and that is almost always the case—the last portion of the interview should include not only an offer of treatment but the formulation and the treatment plan. Based on these ideas, you must negotiate a treatment contract. These topics are covered in subsequent chapters.

Clinical Example: Sally and Julia

To illustrate some of the foregoing ideas, we can look at a sample interview. Sally Skillful, the therapist we met in Chapter One,[6] is meeting a new patient. She is in her private office where her receptionist has just told her the patient has arrived.

Sally steps out into the waiting room. She wears a gray top over dark gray slacks and low heels. She has a blue and green scarf draped loosely around her neck and shoulders. In addition to her engagement and wedding rings, she wears a narrow gold ring set with a garnet on her right ring finger. Julia has dark brown hair and green framed eyeglasses. She is dressed in a brown- and rust-striped shirtwaist dress with a wide black belt and black lace-up shoes. She has a wedding band on her left hand and a red and blue enameled flower pin on her left shoulder.

Sally	Good morning. I'm Sally Skillful. Please come in.
	Sally introduces herself in a neutral fashion: not "Dr. Skillful," not "Sally." She preserves her options on how formal she needs to be with a patient she does not yet know. Most patients would respond to this introduction with later

---

[6]See page 20.

use of Sally's title and last name (Dr. Skillful, Ms. Skillful), but some would now choose a first-name basis. Their choice would reveal something about their expectations and social skills.

Julia   Hi, I'm Julia. (*She follows Sally into the office and takes the chair across from Sally's.*)

Julia responds with just her first name. Sally takes note and wonders if Julia has dependency issues.

Sally   So, what can I do for you?

Sally's receptionist took the telephone referral and her written referral note says only "54-year-old married woman with depression," so Sally does not start by telling Julia what she knows about her.

Julia   I'm having problems in my marriage. I don't know what to do. Should I go? Should I stay? I can't make a decision.

Sally nods encouragingly.

Julia   It all started when Jenny, my youngest, left for college. That was six months ago. My older daughter, Alex, she's a senior, so both girls are gone, and it was just me and Hank. We hadn't been on our own for—over 20 years, I guess—and it's like we didn't know what to say to each other.

Sally frowns slightly and nods again. Her expression is one of concerned understanding.

Julia   So I always get home from work first—we both work at the same place, this Ford dealership—and Hank started going out for drinks with his salesmen. He's the Sales Manager. By the time he gets home, he's drunk, he's had dinner, and he watches TV and goes to bed.

Sally could say, at this point, "It sounds like Hank's having a problem with the girls gone too" (what I describe

	as a "bottom-up" intervention"), but she does not yet know enough to jump in with her own observations that might deflect Julia from her narrative. She could ask about Hank's drinking, to see if he has alcohol dependence, but that would shift the focus away from Julia, who is speaking with some pressure, and Sally wants to let her take the lead at this point.
Sally	Tell me a little more about the problems you and Hank have been having.
	Sally indicates her interest in Julia's problem with an open-ended request for more information.
Julia	It's been going on a long time. I'm not even sure when we started drifting apart. We were both busy with other things. Raising the girls. Work. Less and less sex, and now it's been a really long time. He has a very demanding job. He has sales quotas and all the salesmen. I work every day, but I don't have the kind of pressure he does. I'm just doing the same routine things. I'm just working for the paycheck.
	Sally has said little so far, but Julia's pressured speech is beginning to slow. Sally has two tentative DSM-5 diagnoses: persistent depressive disorder (chronic depression lasting over two years) and adjustment disorder, with depressed mood (depression lasting less than six months).
Sally	So this has all been going on for a good while. How did you decide to come see me?
	Sally combines the "Why here" and "Why now" questions.
Julia	Well, two weeks ago, Hank went to a sales convention, up at that casino, and he was away for five days, and he never called me. So I mentioned to my boss that we were having problems. I was crying at

my desk. And she said she'd heard good things about
you. And when Hank got home, we had a big fight,
and then I decided to call your office.

> *Julia answers both questions (the "Why*
> *now" is Hank's failure to call her and*
> *the "Why here" is the recommendation*
> *from someone in authority). Her boss's*
> *recommendation supports the thera-*
> *peutic alliance.*

Sally   (*nods*) You said before you couldn't make a decision about whether to stay in the marriage. Is that
what you want help with, making that decision?

> *Sally looks for an answer to "What does*
> *she want?"*

Julia   There's just so many things to consider. What
about the girls? What would I do? It's like my mind
is buzzing all the time.

> *The answer is not yet clear, and Julia*
> *seems quite anxious about it. Her speech*
> *pattern has shifted to slower and more*
> *hesitant. Sally wonders if this change re-*
> *flects her depression. Slow speech means*
> *she will get less information during the*
> *time available.*

Sally   Can you tell me a little about yourself? Where you
grew up, your education? What happened before
you were married?

> *Sally decides to come back to the ques-*
> *tion of what she wants at a later point.*
> *She asks an open-ended question and*
> *then adds a little guidance to get more*
> *background.*

Julia   (*settles into the chair for the first time*) I was born in Wyoming, and I grew up there. I went to a community
college in Casper for a business course, but I couldn't
find a full-time job, so I was temping for a few years,
and then I met Hank, and we got married. We moved
here for his job. We had the girls, and after they were

in high school I went back to work. Hank told me there was an opening at the dealership. And I've been there since.

> *This concise summary suggests Julia's memory and cognition are good, but her summary leaves out a lot of information Sally would like to hear about.*

Sally What about your family? Are they back in Wyoming?

> *At this point Sally feels she can be more active, although she still wants to ask these partially open-ended questions. With a more talkative patient, she might say nothing or ask, "Can you tell me more about that?"*

Julia My Mom is. My Dad died a few years back. My sister's there. She's five years older than me, so we weren't real close. She's divorced with three kids. I haven't been back there in a while.

> *The answer raises several topics of interest. Among them: What effect has her father's death had on her relationship with Hank? How does her sister's divorce impact her thinking about a possible separation from Hank? Is she as isolated from her family as this answer suggests?*

Sally What's your Mom like?

> *Sally elects to ask for more information about Julia's mother because Julia's answer seemed to skip over her.*

Julia She's a homebody. Me and my sister were her main job and taking care of the house. About 19–20 years ago, just after I moved east, she got into being born-again. Joined a different church. Now that my Dad's gone, I think that church is her whole life. I'm not much for religion myself. And I don't see her or speak with her so often now, just on birthdays and holidays. We've drifted apart over the years.

> *Again, Sally could intervene by asking if her mother had the same kind of prob-*

lems that Julia has now when she moved away and both Julia and her sister were "out of the nest." Instead, she remains focused on getting to know Julia better and files this observation away for possible future use.

| Sally | How about your social circle here. Do you have close friends? |

Sally looks for evidence of a social support system that might help Julia through her current problems.

| Julia | We socialize—or we did—with people from work, so not much lately. I guess I'm close to my neighbor, Betty, across the street. We're about the same age, and I've gotten to know her pretty well over the years. |

| Sally | What does she think about your situation with Hank? |

Sally wonders if this friend offers a potential social support. With no family and only one friend, she seems somewhat isolated.

| Julia | Betty thinks I should leave him. She says there's nothing there for me anymore. |

| Sally | But you're not sure. Do you think therapy will help you with the decision? |

Sally is still looking for an answer to what Julia wants.

| Julia | I know it's up to me. Suppose I get divorced? What then? I'd still see Hank at work. And what would I do with myself? |

Julia still has no direct answer.

| Sally | So it sounds like it's more than just what to do about the marriage. It's what to do with the rest of your life. |

Perhaps this is what she wants help with?

| Julia | Yes. I'm 54. I can't just start over. |

Maybe it is.

| Sally | Is that how you feel? |

Sally wants to explore this idea.

Julia   I went from my parents' house to living with Hank. I've never been on my own, my whole life. Whenever I think about what to do, I have this thought: I'm no good, and I won't get better.

Sally   Sounds pretty bleak. When did you decide that?

> *Sally has identified an "automatic thought" and wants to clarify Julia's belief system.*

Julia   I don't know. I've felt like this a long time.
Sally   Before you were married?

> *Sally looks for the past history of this negative attitude.*

Julia   No...Well, yes, come to think of it. I can remember in high school I was always pretty down.

Sally   And what does that mean, "I'm no good"?

Julia   It means...I'm not sure what it means. It's just the way I think about myself.

Sally   That's something we need to figure out then. It sounds like a pretty important part of why you feel bad.

> *At this point in the interview, Sally has decided she can treat Julia and she better understands Julia's presenting problem. She has narrowed down the diagnosis to a depressive disorder. She has tentative answers to her three questions, although what exactly Julia "wants" still needs clarification. Depending on Sally's general orientation, she could construct three hypotheses.*
>
> 1. *Psychodynamic: Julia is responding to the loss of her identity as a mother with an "empty nest" depression that resulted from both daughters moving out of the home.*
> 2. *Cognitive-behavioral: Her core belief that she is capable of being a mother*

and nothing else, surfaces in her au-tomatic thought, I'm no good, and I won't get better.

3. *Existential: She is confronted with her increasing isolation as her daugh-ters have left and her husband has lost interest, so that her life now seems without meaning.*

Julia seems to be of average to perhaps above-average intelligence and without cognitive deficits. She is not very psycho-logically minded. Sally wonders about dependency issues but is not ready to ex-plore these yet.

Sally	I'd like to hear a little more about that period of your life after college and before you met Hank. What was that like? What were you like?
	Sally decides to explore her premarital history to see if her current problems are from the marriage or are more general.
Julia	At loose ends. I felt depressed. I was lonely. I had no direction.
Sally	You were depressed. Did it ever get bad enough that you felt suicidal?
	Sally now becomes more active in her assessment. She needs more specific in-formation and a better history.
Julia	No. I was still hopeful.
Sally	How about now? Do you have thoughts about harming yourself? Anything like that?
	Sally checks for current safety issues.
Julia	No, I don't. Not even now.
SALLY	How about the opposite mood? Did you ever have too much energy? Couldn't sleep, ideas all over the place, talking a mile a minute?
	Sally checks for a bipolar pattern.

Julia   (*laughs ruefully*) No, never. That's not me.

Sally   And back then, before Hank, what was going on in your life that was the good part?

> *Sally wonders what long-standing strengths and abilities Julia might have that would help her if she decides to go it alone.*

Julia   Well, I liked temping. There were always new situations, new people. It was kind of an adventure.

> *Sally can explore this issue later at greater length, but she lacks the time in this initial session.*

Sally   And then you met Hank? What was that like?

> *Sally tries to get a better sense of their marriage.*

Julia   I met him at my last temp job, at a dealership in Casper, a place like where I'm working now. He was very confident, a salesman, you know. He took me out to nice restaurants. We had fun. I was surprised when he asked me to marry him, though. I didn't love him, but I thought I wouldn't get another offer. I was never very popular with guys. I thought I wasn't good enough. So when he asked me, I said yes.

> *Julia punctuates this last remark with a "nose wipe" gesture that tells Sally that her feelings for Hank have turned negative even though her words about him seem complimentary.*

Sally   Do you regret that decision now?

> *A key question for the decision about divorce.*

Julia   In some ways I do, but look, it got me my two girls.

> *Again: a topic to explore in more detail later.*

Sally   Okay, and how about earlier in life? What was it like for you growing up?

Julia   I think I was a happy-go-lucky kid. A bit of a tom-
             boy. I liked sports. I played shortstop on our softball
             team. I ran track in the winter. I remember I liked to
             sing. We had a school choir that I was in.

Sally   What about friends?
                          Was Julia always so isolated?

Julia   I had two good friends, girls from the neighbor-
             hood. One family moved away and the other girl
             married a career Marine, so I don't know where she
             is now.

Sally   (*glances at the clock*) So, anything else you want to
             tell me at this point? Anything I should know?

Julia   Nothing I can think of.

Sally   Well, then let me tell you how things look to me so
             far, and then we can talk about what to do about it.

                          On the basis of what she has heard,
                          Sally has put together the following for-
                          mulation and tentative plan: Julia is a
                          54-year-old married woman with mari-
                          tal disharmony who has become de-
                          pressed (or more depressed) because her
                          last child has left home and her life feels
                          empty. The aim of therapy should be to
                          help her find a meaningful life "after
                          motherhood." Therapy objectives should
                          include 1) resolution of marital uncer-
                          tainty, 2) development of new life goals,
                          and 3) increased social support. The
                          therapeutic approach may include cog-
                          nitive, psychodynamic, and existential
                          elements.

Sally   I think you've come to a point in your life where
             you're finishing one phase, the part where you
             raised your girls. They're beginning to make their
             own way now, and they'll need you less than they
             did before.

Julia   Maybe they won't need me at all.

Sally   I doubt that, but wouldn't you feel good about knowing they could build on all the things you've given them over the years?

> *Sally makes a questionable "support-ive" comment but then challenges the negative overgeneralization both as a test of her hypothesis and of the therapeutic approach she hopes to use.*

Julia   I guess so. When you put it that way.

> *Julia's response is noncommittal, an early hint of future resistance.*

Sally   I think what we should try to do in our therapy work is to look for an answer to what you should do with your life at this point. It seems to me that that's the basic question you're facing now. What do you think?

> *Sally advances her idea of the aim of the therapy.*

Julia   I think you're right, but what about me and Hank?

> *Again, Julia agrees but may not have entirely accepted Sally's premise.*

Sally   That's certainly part of what you need to decide, but I don't think that's the whole story. You also need to look beyond the marriage, whatever you decide to do about it, and consider what your personal goals should be. And also, you seem very isolated. It would help to widen your social circle, to have more people in your life than just Hank and the woman across the street.

> *Sally mentions the other two goals she wants to include.*

Julia   I see what you mean.

> *Sally realizes she does not yet have a genuine treatment agreement and that she will probably need to work on it further, but it is the end of today's session.*

Sally   What I'd suggest is that we meet once a week and
               talk about those ideas and see how it goes. But our
               time is up for today, and we have to stop. What
               would you like to do?

Julia   I think I'd like to try it.

We might fault Sally's interview in three respects:

- She touched on a number of topics but did not follow any of them
  through to the point where she fully understood them.
- She tried to cover both past and present history and consequently did
  not get as complete a picture of Julia's present circumstances as she
  might have done.
- She described the therapy work only in vague terms ("talk about those
  ideas") and failed to propose a specific strategy.

As a result, she and Julia have an incomplete treatment contract that
could lead to later problems. Nevertheless, this first interview was successful in that she

1. Began to build the therapeutic alliance, although Julia's depressed
   mood seemed to inhibit her investment in the therapy relationship.
2. Established a working diagnosis.
3. Checked for safety and found no immediate threats.
4. Found answers to the three questions and has a skeletal but adequate history.
5. Decided Julia is suitable for the planned therapy, although some early
   resistance is apparent.
6. Made effective use of the time available and avoided tangential issues and nonrelevant topics.
7. Developed a reasonable initial formulation.
8. Made a start on an agreed-upon plan that will be the basis of the
   treatment contract.

Final Thoughts

The first moments of your initial session with the patient set the tone not
only for the evaluation but sometimes for the entire therapy period. The
initial evaluation is a complex undertaking (Table 4–3). It is further com-

plicated by confrontation with a new patient whom you do not yet understand. In this endeavor, you must

- Establish a therapeutic alliance.
- Decide on a diagnostic impression.
- Gather a useful history.
- Formulate the case.
- Decide whether to offer treatment, and if so,
- Offer a treatment plan.
- Negotiate a treatment contract.

Sometimes, all of these tasks fall neatly into place, but when they do not, some of the work must extend into subsequent sessions. At times—with a patient with a difficult personality disorder, for example—negotiations can become a central focus of the treatment. Most of the time, fortunately, these various efforts can be successfully concluded within a reasonable time frame. Perhaps the biggest challenge is the need to maintain focus on the assessment process and not let yourself be distracted by temptations to engage in premature therapy interventions. As I discuss in Chapter Six, successful planning requires a top-down approach in which the choice of specific therapy techniques is at the end of the planning process.

TABLE 4–3. Assessment: goals and requirements

Stage	Goals	Requirements
Early	Therapeutic alliance, provisional diagnosis	Bonding skills, deductive analysis
Middle	Relevant history, mental status, safety assessment, decision to treat	Personal and historical information, three questions, tentative hypotheses, suitability
Late	Formulation, treatment plan, treatment contract	Inductive analysis, top-down decisions, negotiation

Key Points

- The initial interview is a unique opportunity to begin the therapeutic alliance.
- The major goals for the interview are:
  - ➤ Obtain a history and diagnosis.
  - ➤ Assess the patient's need and suitability for treatment.
  - ➤ Decide whether to treat the patient.
  - ➤ Formulate the case.
  - ➤ Construct the treatment plan.
  - ➤ Negotiate a treatment contract.
- A semistructured interview is the best format to accomplish these tasks.
- Important questions are the following:
  - ➤ Why did the patient come here?
  - ➤ Why did the patient come now?
  - ➤ What does the patient want?
- Making and testing hypotheses is a useful way to begin the formulation of the case.

CHAPTER
FIVE

What Is a Formulation?

> Anyone who has ever attempted a pure scientific or philosophical thought knows how one can hold a problem momentarily in one's mind and apply all one's powers of concentration to piercing through it, and how it will dissolve and escape and you find that what you are surveying is a blank.
>
> *John Maynard Keynes*

> It's tough to make predictions, especially about the future.
>
> *Yogi Berra*

Introduction

In the final portion of your initial interview, your evaluation should have gathered enough history, and the right kind of history, to formulate the case. A formulation is an explanation of how and why the patient developed the problems you propose to treat. It usually has three components:

1. A brief case description with the demographic identifiers, the presenting problem, and a formal diagnosis
2. Relevant history: central issues, hypotheses, and cause-and-effect connections
3. A narrative summary

The second and third components are sometimes combined. If your initial assessment allows you to construct a complete formulation, you will be in a strong position to

- Understand the patient.
- Develop an effective therapeutic alliance.
- Decide on the best treatment approach.
- Negotiate a treatment contract with the patient.
- Begin treatment with a solid foundation and clear objectives.

As an example of a complete formulation, consider the following short example:

> David is a 25-year-old single male graduate student who presents with a three-month history of depressed mood, insomnia, anorexia, and suicidal ideation without a plan. The diagnosis is major depressive disorder. The onset occurred after his fiancée broke their engagement. A previous romantic breakup when he was 17 was followed by a similar, although milder, episode that resolved without treatment. His father died when he was 11. His mother and maternal grandmother have had recurrent depressions. In summary, this 25-year-old man has a history of recurrent depression precipitated by loss of a close relationship in the context of early loss of his father and a family predisposition to depressive illness.

The first sentence identifies the patient and the presenting symptoms. The second gives a diagnosis. The four sentences that follow contain the relevant history on which to base the cause-and-effect hypothesis in the final, summary sentence. Based solely on these few facts, we could imagine a treatment plan that combined medication and cognitive-behavioral therapy (CBT).

You might think you could have reached the same treatment decisions with only the information in the first two sentences. In that case, your conclusion would be based on the diagnosis alone, and in this straightforward example, it would be a reasonable choice: medication and CBT for depression. Simple enough, although what the focus of therapy would be remains unclear. The information in the midsection of the formulation would no doubt emerge in the course of the therapy and would be consistent with the selected approach.

The failings of this shortcut arise, however, when we think of more complicated case presentations and other diagnostic categories. To review the problems with psychiatric diagnosis mentioned in the last chapter:

- At our present level of knowledge, diagnosis is almost entirely based on observed phenomena, the ones listed as criteria in each of the categories in our current classification.
- Specific etiologies, the kind that underpin almost all medical diagnoses, are at present sadly lacking in the mental health field.

- Political and cultural considerations sometimes influence psychiatric taxonomy.
- The distinctions between diagnostic categories can be arbitrary, such as the separation between dissociative disorders and traumatic stress disorders, or between traumatic stress disorders and anxiety disorders.
- At this stage in our knowledge of the brain, the scientific method does not often provide a path to diagnostic accuracy. Future neurophysiological studies will undoubtedly allow us to better define the psychotic disorders, affective disorders, and other major illnesses.
- Behavioral disorders will probably be the last to yield to brain research.

As a result of these deficiencies, the mere diagnosis alone will not usually tell us what to treat or what treatment to use. In fact, the same treatments are often applied to patients diagnosed with many of the disorders in DSM. Specific, diagnosis-based treatment remains an unrealized goal.

Furthermore, a patient's history will often not fit neatly and completely into a single diagnostic category. In the earlier brief example of David, the depressed graduate student,

- Our patient may have difficulties with interpersonal relationships, especially romantic ones, that are not captured by the diagnosis of "major depression."
- He may have problems with his emotional development, due to the loss of a parent, that also fall outside that category.
- Further history might show us that he is struggling with an issue of adult independence that is reflected in his status as a graduate student.

None of these potential therapeutic topics can be imagined merely by knowing his diagnostic label, and it may turn out, as we get to know him better, that CBT is not the best approach.

A Neglected Exercise

With all its advantages for treatment planning, you would think that case formulation would be a high priority goal and a natural result of the initial consultation. Unfortunately, the opposite seems to be true. Although frequently praised in texts, and recognized in many published treatment methodologies, formulation appears to be as widely ignored as it is recommended.

One reason for the lack of attention to formulation is that, to some practitioners, it may not seem to have any real purpose. The function of a formulation is to provide the basis for a treatment plan. But what if you do not intend to make a plan? If you have only one treatment skill, and you intend to use it for every patient, your requirement of a treatment plan is much reduced. True, you might want to decide what the purpose of your treatment might be—its ultimate outcome—but you may feel you do not need to identify it. As the saying goes, if your only tool is a hammer, every problem looks like a nail.

- If you employ CBT as outlined by Aaron Beck, you know you will identify automatic thoughts and work on the core beliefs they reflect.
- If you are a Freudian psychoanalyst, you expect to allow the patient to free-associate until a transference develops that you can then analyze.

Never mind that neither Beck nor Freud would begin without a formulation, plenty of contemporary therapists might feel comfortable knowing they have a procedure to follow and not bother with trying to understand the origins of the patient's difficulties. This limited approach may not be as successful as one rooted in an understanding of the patient, but it is certainly easier.

To be a successful practitioner, however, you need an array of psychotherapy skills. Sometimes this approach means

- You combine elements of different methodologies to deal with the varied problems of one case. For example, you might start with a psychodynamic plan but use a behavioral approach for the patient's insomnia.
- You use treatments in parallel to deal with different therapy goals. For example, you might employ a cognitive strategy for a patient's depressed mood but use a transactional method for interpersonal problems.

In other words, instead of limiting yourself to a hammer, you need an assortment of tools to take on a variety of treatment projects.

A second reason that formulation is underutilized may be inadequate training. Just like the textbooks, training programs may give lip service to this part of the curriculum but fail to adequately instruct their students in how to do it. Supervisors and other instructors, perhaps listening to a trainee's clinical presentation, may accept a simple summary of the case as a good-enough formulation. As a result, you may emerge from your training program not only without an appreciation of the significance of a formulation but also without the preparation needed to carry it out.

The most important reason for the neglect of formulation, however, may be that it can pose a formidable intellectual challenge. Case formulation confronts the therapist with the need to use an unfamiliar type of logic: inductive reasoning. This process requires that you move from the specific to the general, from the concrete to the abstract, from a set of data to the one category into which they all fit.

Inductive Versus Deductive Logic

Much of current healthcare training and experience centers not on inductive reasoning but on its opposite, deduction. Deductive logic requires you to draw a single conclusion from all the data available, from the general to the specific. To make a diagnosis, a common deductive exercise, the more information you have, the easier it is to find the single category into which it all fits. In the previous example, simply knowing David had a depressed mood would not narrow the diagnosis, since it is not specific to "major depression." Include insomnia, anorexia, and suicidal thoughts, and major depression looks more certain. With the addition of a prior history of depression, your confidence in the diagnosis improves further. *In deductive reasoning the more data you have, the easier it is to reach the correct conclusion.*

With inductive reasoning, however, the opposite is true (Table 5–1). The more data you have, the more difficult it is to find the single category that encompasses all of it. For instance, consider the mental status exam question: what is the same about a chair and a table? Best answer: they are both furniture. You must be familiar with the characteristics of the two objects, but you do not require a knowledge of wood glues, carpentry, or the history of dining. If you add to those two items a set of dishes and a pot roast, you need a more abstract concept: perhaps, "my last night's dinner." What about: twelve chairs, a circular table, a set of dishes, a pot roast, Sir Thomas Malory, and a broadsword? That could be the Round Table in the legend of King Arthur. Not only is that solution more abstract yet, but it requires additional knowledge: the history of England and a familiarity with its literature.

Sometimes, no sensible answer is possible. Take the riddle from Alice in Wonderland. The Mad Hatter asks Alice: why is a raven like a writing

TABLE 5–1. Logical types

Deductive	Inductive
From the general to the specific	From the particular to the general
The more data the easier	The more data the greater the difficulty
Reduces complexity	Multiplies complexity
Familiar medical model logic	Unfamiliar nonlinear logic
Result: single common label	Result: multifaceted explanation
Training program staple	Training may ignore

desk? There is no correct answer: Lewis Carroll was asked about it, and he said so. In spite of Carroll's assertion, people have tried to find a category into which the two would fit for the last 150 years. Sometimes a patient's history feels the same way: no category contains all the data. Sometimes, the effort to apply inductive logic fails. In taking a history from a patient

- You are often confronted with an increasing mass of disparate information.
- Historical data do not all fit neatly into a single narrative but fall within separate areas.
- You can access only a limited portion of the history and the pieces will not always fit together.
- As you learn more about the patient, the struggle to reach an inductive conclusion becomes more and more difficult.

Formulation Simplified: The Use of Categories

The difficulty posed by the need for inductive reasoning to formulate a case can be at least partially overcome if we can narrow the choices and provide a single framework, a predefined category, for understanding each particular patient. Such a shortcut would require that we define a set of (seven) categories for the most common patient presentations. We can then choose a single category for each patient. Finally, we can use the framework provided by that category to organize the patient's history.

The advantage of a set of categories is that it bypasses the inductive first step in the formulation process and substitutes a deductive conclusion. With this approach the more information you have, the easier it is to select the right "diagnostic" answer.

- Most case histories will fall within one of the seven general groups outlined below.
- Once a category is selected, its own characteristics suggest the cause-and-effect connections that together will create a coherent rationale for treatment decisions.
- These connections, along with the relevant points of the history, can then be combined into the final formulation.

STEP ONE: SELECT A CATEGORY

Grouping patient presentations into a common set requires a broader and more inclusive collection of data than that used to identify individual diagnoses. The criteria listed for an individual diagnosis not only reflect its observed characteristics but also attempt to separate and differentiate it from similar or related conditions. This effort is part of the deductive process. Formulation categories, by contrast, are based on shared characteristics, the common ground that links the members of each category with all the others. This grouping represents the end result of a prior inductive process. For example, two diagnoses within the dissociative category—dissociative identity disorder and posttraumatic stress disorder (PTSD)—are linked by the common etiological factor of trauma. In this exercise, the initial inductive step—the particular to the general—is already provided (the inclusive feature is *trauma*) so that the clinician can more easily find the inclusive "label" needed to begin the formulation process.

The seven categories listed below do not follow the standard diagnostic classifications. Rather they are groupings of common problem areas, each of which includes similar clinical presentations. With that foundation, here are the seven categories[1] (Table 5–2):

1. Biological
2. Developmental
3. Dissociative
4. Situational
5. Transactional

---

[1] A useful mnemonic, formed by the first letters of each category, is BDD-STEP.

6. Existential
7. Psychodynamic

Discussion and examples of each category are provided later in this chapter.

This classification does not include personality disorders, other than those interpersonal consequences noted as "type two" in the transactional category (see below). Although we call these "disorders," they are really exaggerations of normal groups of traits, somewhat arbitrarily put together. A personality disorder diagnosis highlights a specified group of traits, but in clinical practice it is much more common to see people with the characteristics of two or three or more of the various divisions. We all have personalities and share many of the traits that are listed under these headings. To a greater or lesser, but still acceptable, degree, we are narcissistic, avoidant, obsessive, dependent, and the rest. The patients we place in one of the seven formulation categories will also have some of these traits, and they may be factors that contribute to their difficulties. In the past these problems were relegated to Axis II in the DSM system, a recognition of their subsidiary but pervasive influence.

It is unusual for someone who fits the criteria for a personality disorder to seek therapy for the troublesome traits that qualify them for that diagnosis. You rarely encounter a chief complaint of "I'm too narcissistic …avoidant…obsessive…dependent." Instead it is the secondary effects of those qualities that impel people into treatment: "I'm too thin-skinned …too shy…too perfectionistic…too sensitive to rejection." And even these complaints are, in turn, secondary to less self-referenced problems: "I can't get along with people…I'm too nervous…People tell me my standards are too high…nobody loves me." Maladaptive traits are more usefully acknowledged when treatment goals are being set and need not be considered at the *initial* stage of grouping the patient's problems into one of these seven step-one categories.

STEP TWO: IDENTIFY CAUSATIONS

The human brain is hard-wired to look for patterns. Whether we want to or not, we cannot perceive a set of facts without trying to fit them together into whatever order we can in our effort to try to make sense of the world around us. This tendency can lead us into bigotry or even delusional ideation, or it can be the basis of a new scientific breakthrough. So, as we listen to and observe a patient, even in a first meeting, we cannot help but try to find the pattern that brings order to the history and "explains" the

TABLE 5–2. The seven formulation categories

Category	Description	Example
Biological	Disorders with a known or likely organic substrate	Schizoaffective disorder
Developmental	Problems arising from a failed transition in a phase of maturation	Identity crisis
Dissociative	Responses to trauma, abuse, or neglect	Posttraumatic stress disorder
Situational	Stress-related symptoms caused by inadequate coping skills	Adjustment disorder with anxiety
Transactional	Impaired social function stemming from interpersonal difficulties	Marital crisis
Existential	Anxiety and despair related to meaninglessness, isolation, or death	Depression associated with life-threatening illness
Psychodynamic	Irrational behavior reflecting intrapsychic conflict related to earlier life problems	Hypochondriasis

problems the patient is having. Our need for this explanation is so strong that we are at risk of drawing incorrect conclusions just so that we have conclusions and not a disorganized muddle of unrelated facts.

In finding this pattern, we are naturally inclined to use a template provided by the theory associated with a particular methodology. That could involve a cognitive explanation or psychodynamic ideas or some other contemporary theory. Remember that those same facts in the past would have been ascribed to supernatural forces and in the future—who knows?—may be explained by neurochemical reactions. As Jerome Frank suggested (see Chapter Two[2]), one explanation may be as good as an-

---

[2]See pages 37–38.

other, constituting the "myth" that promotes psychological healing. The advantage to organizing the history into a theoretical framework to find a pattern in the mix of facts is that it allows us to create a formulation.

In order to decide on *what* to treat (regardless of *how* you will do so), it is important to understand what brought about the patient's current condition. In other words, based on your observation of the patient and the history you have obtained so far, you can construct one or more cause-and-effect hypotheses. The "effects" with which you are concerned are the evidence of the patient's problems, the signs and symptoms of the disorder. The "causes" of those particular effects are the past and present influences responsible for those symptoms. For example, if you see a soldier with PTSD that followed a battlefield attack that killed everyone but him, you could reasonably conclude that his combat experience was the cause of his symptoms.

Logical Errors

Because you are programmed by biology and training to find patterns in a patient's history, your cause-and-effect reasoning is exposed to the risk of logical error. There are many fallacies in formal logic, but two types that occur frequently in clinical assessment are the *cum hoc* and the *post hoc* errors.

The Cum Hoc Ergo Propter Hoc[3] Fallacy

This error can be summarized as: *correlation is not causation*. If you see two events, A and B, that occur together, then they are correlated, but you cannot assume that A caused B or that B caused A. They may be unconnected. They may both have been caused by another event, C. Here are two examples:

1. All the boys (A) in the class (B) have the measles (C). Missing data: we do not know whether the class is all boys or whether it is coed. What are the cause-and-effect relationships among these three facts?
    - Does being a boy cause measles? No, it is merely a correlation. (A and C are correlated.)
    - Does measles cause children to become boys? No, again, just a correlation. (A and C are correlated.)
    - Does the measles virus cause measles only in boys? No. If the class is all boys, no girls were exposed. (B and C are correlated.)

---

[3]"With this, therefore because of this."

- Even if the class was coed and only boys were ill, no cause-and-effect relationship has been established between sex and illness, not by these facts alone. (B and C are still just correlated.)
- Does being in the class cause boys to get measles? Probably, yes; they infected one another. Contagion by physical proximity is a cause of measles. (B and C are cause and effect.)

2. John is depressed (A). John's wife, Mary, is depressed (B). John lost his job (C), and he and his wife had to move out of their home (D). How are these facts related?

    - Is John's depression caused by Mary's depression? No, they are merely correlated. (A and B are correlated.)
    - Is John's unemployment (C) related to the loss of their home (D)? Yes. (C is the cause of D.)
    - Are both their depressions connected to D, their loss of their home? Yes, perhaps. (D may be the cause of both A and B.)

Notice in both examples that the true causes can only be conjectured because too little information is available for certainty. Even without a logical error, the accuracy of a deduction may be uncertain because not enough of the relevant facts are known.

- The boys may have caught the measles from a birthday party they all attended.
- No girls caught the measles because they all had had measles before and they were immune.
- Perhaps John had had several episodes of depression before his job loss, and Mary became depressed by the debilitating effect that John's problems had on their relationship.
- Perhaps John and Mary had to move out of their home because of a fire.

The Post Hoc Ergo Propter Hoc[4] Fallacy

This error can be summarized as: *temporal connection is not causation.* This fallacy occurs when the mere circumstance that one event follows another prompts the conclusion that the earlier event caused the later. A occurs and then B occurs; therefore, A caused B. This error is especially likely when only limited information is available, hiding the real causes of the observed results. Two examples again:

---

[4]"After this, therefore because of this."

1. Every time John stops at a railroad crossing (A) when the gates are down (B), a train goes by (C).

   - Does John cause the train to pass the crossing? No. (A is not the cause of C.)
   - Does lowering the gates cause the train to cross the roadway? No. (B is not a cause of C.)

   In fact, the approach of the train (C) causes the gates to lower (B). The lowered barrier causes John to stop (A): C is the cause of B and B is the cause of A.

2. John became depressed (A) after he lost his job (B).

   - Did getting fired cause his depression? No, probably not. (B is not the cause of A.)

   In fact, other (unknown) factors could have caused it: perhaps John was fired (B) because of poor performance (C), which in turn was caused by the onset of Parkinson's disease (D) that was the actual cause of his depression: D then caused both A and C, and C caused B.

   Once again, the error occurs because of a paucity of information. In the first example, it is ignorance of how the train gates work; in the second, it is an incomplete medical history.

Successive Approximations

Even though your initial interview has provided only a limited history and an incomplete set of facts, you must nevertheless form hypotheses that organize the available data to establish causation. It helps to keep in mind the risk of logical error that results from limited data, and to avoid fallacious conclusions, but simply having a hypothesis is an advantage. It provides a framework for your ongoing attention to the history and your subsequent observations. Your initial conclusions can only be an approximation. At a later stage, when you have more information, you can revise your hypotheses or create new ones. Even if your original, and your subsequent, explanations are incomplete and subject to further revision, your successive approximations will move you closer and closer to a better understanding of your patient.

A useful format for these hypotheses is a statement using "because …" or "because of…" as a link between your observations and your explanations. In the case of David, the depressed graduate student cited earlier, we had the following summary:

David is a 25-year-old single male graduate student who presents with a three-month history of depressed mood, insomnia, anorexia, and suicidal ideation without a plan. The diagnosis is major depressive disorder. The onset occurred after his fiancée broke their engagement. A previous romantic breakup when he was 17 was followed by a similar although milder episode that resolved without treatment. His father died when he was 11. His mother and maternal grandmother have had recurrent depressions.

Even with this very limited information we can construct the following hypotheses, based on the data and our knowledge of major depression:

1. David is vulnerable to depression *because of* a family history of mood disorders. (We know that major depression tends to run in families.)
2. The depression is occurring at this point in time *because of* the loss of his fiancée. (We know that depression is often precipitated by loss.)
3. He is particularly sensitive to loss *because of* earlier losses: his father died when he was 11 and a prior romantic breakup was followed by an earlier depressive episode. (We know that a history of early losses increases vulnerability.)

Contrast the format used here with the way we described our conclusions in the original case description:

In summary, this 25-year-old man has a history of recurrent depression precipitated by loss of a close relationship in the context of early loss of his father and a family predisposition to depressive illness.

The information and the conclusions do not differ, but the *because of* format will lead more readily to the treatment goals we need to plan a course of treatment. *Because* statements more clearly answer the *why* of each piece of data:

- *Why* is David vulnerable to depression? *Because* he has a positive family history.
- *Why* is he depressed now? *Because* his fiancée broke the engagement.
- *Why* is he sensitive to loss? *Because* of losses earlier in his life.

Although at this point, with limited data, we cannot tell for sure if these deductions are the result of correlation and temporal errors (the *cum hoc* and *post hoc* fallacies), we at least have a starting point for our formulation. Further exploration may yield additional relevant facts that will alter our ideas, or the new information may strengthen them as we learn more about David and his responses to those events.

Ultimate, Intermediate, and Proximal Causes

It is also useful to consider how closely linked are the events we want to connect by causation. An event may have an ultimate cause, one or more intermediate causes, and a proximal cause. Consider the rock wall at the edge of a highway, created when the road was cut through a hillside. If a piece of rock breaks off and falls onto the tarmac:

- The *ultimate* cause is tectonic plate movement associated with continental drift that pushed the earth's crust up to form the original hill.
- An *intermediate* cause is the excavation of the hill during highway construction that exposed the rock wall to the elements.
- An *intermediate* cause is the weathering effect of rain and cycles of freezing and heating that over the years produced cracks and fissures in the rock face.
- An *intermediate* cause is the vibrations created by the passing cars and trucks that eventually fractured and loosened the rock.
- The *proximate* cause is the disruption produced by a single heavily loaded tractor-trailer that rumbled past and released the force that dislodged the rock.

The first four causes explain the potential for the falling rock, but only the final, proximate cause accounts for the presence of that particular rock on the roadway. We cannot alter the proximate cause: the rock has already fallen. If we wanted to protect drivers from this danger (our "treatment plan"), we would look for an intermediate cause. We might, for example, recommend that the road be closed to all trucks over two tons. As in this example, most treatment plans are concerned with an intermediate cause.

An example from human behavior is the "epidemic" of rape on college campuses across the country. The prevalence of sexual assault on college women (including the rape statistics) is reported to be (at least) as high as 20%. Other reports suggest that a disproportionately high percentage of the rapes are committed by football players, a group that enjoys enhanced status and privilege and who represent an important source of income and prestige for the colleges. It is also alleged that college authorities and even law enforcement are reluctant to prosecute football players and may shield them from the consequences of their crimes. What causation hypotheses can we develop from these allegations?

- The *ultimate* cause of the rapes is the Darwinian imperative for males to seek the widest possible distribution of their DNA by impregnating as many females as possible. A related factor is the evolution of sexual dimorphism: human males are larger and more powerful than human females, and this difference is especially true of football players, who are selected, in part, because of their size.

- An *intermediate* cause is that privileged status in social groups produces entitlement and increased power, and consequently the high social status of football players may lead them to feel "above the law."
- An *intermediate* cause is that both males and females in this age group, late adolescence, have not yet matured to fully develop good judgment. Instead, they are less able to foresee the consequences of their behavior and to control their impulses.
- An *intermediate* cause is the separation from family and community when students leave home to attend college that both encourages them to express their new-found independence in high-risk behavior and deprives them of social support and protection.
- An *intermediate* cause is the use of alcohol and other drugs that reduce social inhibitions in both football players and college women, including the overuse of alcohol and drugs that may render women unable to withhold consent or to resist sexual assault.
- An *intermediate* cause is the betrayal of women who report a rape by college administration and law enforcement personnel. Administrators, prosecutors, defense attorneys, and the courts may all fail to credit the victim's statements, and punishment of perpetrators, if any, is often trivial compared with crimes of similar severity.
- A *proximal* cause (not the only one) is lust.

Based on these hypotheses, what should colleges do to combat campus rape?

- They cannot change the ultimate cause, the effects of evolution on the behavior of large, powerful, privileged males.
- They cannot alter biological development. Impulsive judgment and increased risk taking among college-age men and women will yield only to future growth and maturation.
- Nor can they eliminate the proximal cause, lust, since it is built into the human psyche.

If we think of the colleges as "therapists" and the students as "patients," what "treatment plans" could the *colleges* undertake? They could take one or both of these measures that would attempt to alter the antecedents of the behavior:

- Because the football culture increases sexual assault, they could attempt to alter the college culture and put student safety ahead of the money and prestige of the football program.
- Because substance abuse is a significant factor in sexual assaults, they could ban the use of alcohol and drugs from campus.

Neither of these interventions seems apt to occur and would be unlikely to succeed if tried. Instead of a change in the college environment, an alternative approach would focus on and attempt to modify intermediate causes of *student* behavior:

- Because students are insufficiently aware of the dangers, colleges could institute proactive measures to educate incoming students about the risk of sexual assaults.
- Because students do not connect alcohol use with unsafe behavior, colleges could educate students about the dangers posed by alcohol and drug use.
- Because social isolation increases vulnerability, colleges could attempt to replicate the family and community protections of the home environment. For example, they could set up safeguards, such as a "buddy system," for women (especially, new students) to look out for and protect one another.

Note, too, that the second set of interventions depends on collaboration between the colleges and their students and that it focuses on student behavior—that is, behavior changes in students—rather than futile efforts to alter the unsafe environment. To continue our analogy with individual therapy: our efforts to ameliorate our patient's problems must be focused on what behaviors *they* can change, rather than on changes in other people or in their social environment.

When we assess a patient for therapy, we are often confronted by similar hierarchies of causation. Just as with the examples of fallen rock and rape on campuses, we usually cannot change ultimate and proximal behaviors. Almost always we must choose one or more intermediate problem areas on which to focus our therapeutic efforts. For example, if we look again at the depression of our graduate student, David:

- The ultimate cause is the genetic predisposition he appears to have inherited from his maternal line.
- An intermediate cause is the developmental disruption created by his father's death when he was 11.

- An intermediate cause is the prior loss he suffered at age 17 when his girlfriend ended their relationship.
- The proximal cause is the loss he incurred when his fiancée broke their engagement.

Again, we cannot change the ultimate and proximal factors: his genetic predisposition and the decision of his fiancée. Thus, our treatment plan would not include genetic counseling or a discussion of strategies for him to reunite with his fiancée. Both of these measures would waste therapy time and divert his energies from more productive areas. Our best chance to help him is to concentrate on the intermediate causes: the effect of past losses on his present behavior. We could propose that he explore the impact of his father's absence on his adolescence and the parallels of his current feelings about the broken engagement with the consequences of his breakup in high school. Our recognition of the differential effects of this series of behavioral "causes" allows us to select the more promising avenues of therapeutic work and to construct a more effective treatment plan.

Ultimate causes have a seductive appeal. Their promise of an inclusive explanation and of complete understanding is misleading. They tempt us to a reductionist approach to formulation. For example, confronted with a man who seduces many women (A) but avoids commitment to a long-term relationship (B), we may conclude he is acting out an oedipal conflict or that he suffers from Peter Pan Syndrome or some other global judgment. Although we might have identified an ultimate cause of his behavior towards women,

- Our abstract conclusion will not provide us with a workable treatment approach.
- Our use of the ultimate cause in his treatment will, at best, elicit only an intellectual response, but no change in behavior.

Any useful evidence will be found in his concrete, everyday actions, emotions, habits and ideas. We might learn, for instance, that after his initial "conquest" he becomes impotent (C). To say his erectile dysfunction (ED) occurs *because* of oedipal conflict would be unjustified. In logical terms, we have a *post hoc* fallacy: his childhood fantasy (A) does not automatically cause his adult behaviors (B) and (C). Instead, we might find a whole history of negative experiences with women more closely linked with his current behavior. We might even find that

- He has early diabetes, an organic cause of ED.
- The ED itself provokes anticipatory anxiety and consequent humiliation, and
- It is these painful feelings that determine his behavior toward women.
- He breaks off relationships because of ED but continues to date in the hope that his ED will improve with a different partner. (C is the cause of B, and B is the cause of A.)

Almost always, the intermediate causes will determine what we should treat and where to focus our efforts.

STEP THREE: ORGANIZE THE SUMMARY

The final step is to organize the patient's history into a format that provides a foundation for planning a course of treatment. In contrast to our original summary of David's case, we might now say:

> In summary, this 25-year-old man has a history of recurrent depression. He is now depressed *because of* a broken engagement. He is predisposed to depression *because of* a positive maternal family history and *because of* the earlier loss of his father and of a high school girlfriend.

Sometimes, as here, the causation statements and the summary statement can be merged. The statements of causation will now provide a foundation for an effective treatment plan.

The Seven Categories: Discussion

This section offers a brief examination of the types of clinical conditions that fit into the formulation categories in order to give a general sense of what kinds of problems should be included in each group. With experience, you should be able to size up your patient's presentation and decide where it fits. In clinical situations that seem to have elements of different categories, your decision should be guided by which category provides the most useful basis for treatment planning.

BIOLOGICAL

In this category would fall those disorders that have been connected, at least tentatively, to a neurophysiological substrate. Included here are not only the obvious conditions, such as the dementias, but also those in which behavior seems to arise from a problem originating in the anatomy and biochemistry of the brain. These conditions comprise the schizophrenias and other psychotic disorders, bipolar and other affective disorders, and disorders arising from substance abuse. Although many of these conditions are susceptible to medication, the simple fact that a medication could be prescribed does not automatically place a disorder in this category, because psychiatric medications

- Are nonspecific, as when, for example "antidepressants" are used to treat "anxiety disorders."
- Are often prescribed to control symptoms rather than to treat the underlying disease.
- Are sometimes used in novel or "off-label" ways, thanks in part to the unceasing efforts of the drug companies to broaden the market for their products.

Table 5–3 contains a list of DSM-5 disorders that fall into the biological category. Although a majority of the disorders listed are associated with a physiological disturbance, some members of the group lack this connection. Everything that happens in the brain, of course, has a biochemical substrate, even if we do not yet know what it is, so this list is valid only for the purpose of constructing a formulation. Reversal or amelioration of the biological problems will be one of the treatment goals of the planned therapy, but usually not the only goal. For example, to revisit the case of David, the graduate student with the broken engagement, our treatment plan might include both an antidepressant medication and a psychodynamic exploration of his vulnerability to loss.

DEVELOPMENTAL

With this category we leave the DSM-5 taxonomy and look instead to the phases of maturation in the human life cycle. We are born into a "family of origin." From infancy we progress through childhood into adolescence, become young adults who may form a new family (the "family of procreation"), and pursue a career, working either within the home (for example, child-rearing) or outside in a business, a trade, or a profession. Our child-rearing days end as our offspring become adults or our career ends in retirement, and we must adjust again. Later, we make a final maturation to old age and then confront the end of life. The transitions between these maturational phases are often periods of psychological difficulty, as we struggle to leave one era behind and take up the

TABLE 5–3.	DSM-5 diagnostic groups with likely "biological" foundations

Neurodevelopmental disorders

Schizophrenia spectrum and other psychotic disorders

Bipolar and related disorders

Depressive disorders*

Feeding and eating disorders*

Elimination disorders

Sleep-wake disorders*

Sexual dysfunctions*

Gender dysphoria

Substance-related and addictive disorders

Neurocognitive disorders

Medication-induced movement disorders

*Some members of this category may not have a "biological" basis.

challenges of the next. Sometimes the tasks inherent in a particular phase prove too much to handle, and we can become stuck at a developmental level that, chronologically, we should have already completed. When patients present with either these transitional difficulties or the inability to cope with a developmental task, they can be placed in this category.

One useful scheme for these phases is provided by Erik Erikson[5] and outlined in Figure 5–1. For each of his eight "stages of man," Erikson defines the task and the consequences of failing to master it. For example, the task in adolescence is to form a new identity, separate from the role of child in the family of origin, and prepare to enter adulthood. If a young person cannot separate from the family in this way, he or she will suffer from "identity diffusion," a condition marked by anxiety, fluctuating emotions, and uncertainty about personal attributes. The person's identity remains unsettled, and, in popular terminology, he or she suffers "an identity crisis."

---

[5]Erikson EH: *Identity and the Life Cycle* (Psychological Issues Series, Monograph 1). New York, International Universities Press, 1959.

I. Infancy	Trust vs. Mistrust						
II. Early Childhood		Autonomy vs. Shame, Doubt					
III. Play Age			Initiative vs. Guilt				
IV. School Age				Industry vs. Inferiority			
V. Adolescence					Identity vs. Identity Diffusion		
VI. Young Adult						Intimacy vs. Isolation	
VII. Adulthood							Generativity vs. Self-Absorption	
VIII. Mature Age								Integrity vs. Disgust, Despair

FIGURE 5–1. Erikson's eight stages.

Source. Adapted from Erikson EH: *Identity and the Life Cycle* (Psychological Issues Series, Monograph 1). New York, International Universities Press, 1959.

CLINICAL EXAMPLE: A MAN UNWILLING TO FACE THE NEXT PHASE OF HIS LIFE (ERIKSON'S STAGE VI: INTIMACY VERSUS ISOLATION)

Dennis is a 25-year-old lawyer who has doubts about his upcoming wedding to Dorothy, a woman he has known for five years. He wants to break the engagement, but a friend convinced him to see a therapist before he made his decision. He is afraid to limit himself to just one relationship ("I'm too young to get married," "How do I know she's the right one?"), he does not want to have a child and start a family ("I'm not ready for that kind of responsibility"), and he worries that it will impact his bond with his parents ("She's not as close to them as I'd like"). These anxieties have resulted in insomnia, a weight loss of twelve pounds, and increasing irritability with his fiancée. He resents her enthusiasm about planning the wedding. He hesitates to break the engagement, however, because he still loves her.

It is hard to see how any hypothesis other than a developmental one would allow us to understand the problem Dennis faces. There is certainly no biological basis for it and no standard diagnostic classification. (We need *some* diagnosis, of course, and "adjustment disorder" will have to do, inadequate as it is, because we want to bill his third-party payer.) Some might question whether Dennis has a "psychiatric disorder," but his behavior is abnormal: insomnia, anorexia leading to weight loss, and inappropriate irritability. In fact, he himself defines his situation as abnormal because he recognizes the ambivalence and his conflicted motives and because he accepts his friend's recommendation to see a therapist. It would not be unusual to encounter a patient like Dennis in a general psychotherapy practice.

Dollard and Miller described the ambivalence an engaged couple faces as an example of an approach-avoidance conflict.[6] When the couple become engaged, the "approach" feelings are high and, with the wedding far off, the "avoidance" worries are low. As the wedding date nears, however, doubt, uncertainty, and anxiety increase and the positive benefits of marriage fade in value (Figure 5–2). If the two lines on the graph cross before the wedding date (avoidance becomes stronger than approach), the marriage will not occur. To prevent this outcome, society interposes a series of events that strengthen the couple's commitment:

---

[6]Dollard J, Miller NE: *Personality and Psychotherapy: An Analysis in Terms of Learning, Thinking, and Culture.* New York, McGraw-Hill, 1950.

- They announce the decision to their families, creating an expectation they feel obligated to fulfill.
- The groom buys an engagement ring, often a significant monetary investment.
- They tell their friends, who plan a bridal shower and a bachelor party, so that now they are under a social obligation.
- They book the church and a reception hall, buy flowers, hire a caterer, and print and send out invitations—all steps that increase their financial (and social) investment.

All these events make it increasingly difficult to reverse their decision. The "universal" reluctance to take this step implied by the social and cultural forces employed to encourage it suggests that Dennis's problem is not unusual. What is different—and what makes the problem a potential therapy case—is that these external forces are failing, as Dennis himself recognizes.

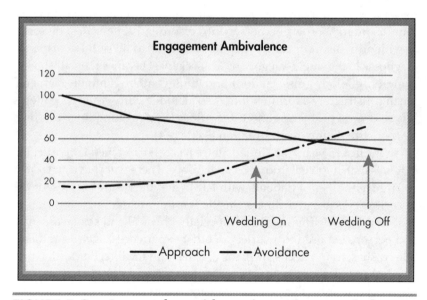

FIGURE 5–2. Approach-avoidance in getting married.

The developmental model is useful in that it can generate cause-and-effect hypotheses that we would need to plan an effective course of treatment. We can hypothesize that

- The negative (avoidance) factors are strengthened by whatever unresolved issues Dennis still has to overcome.

- These unresolved problems include
  - ➤ A reluctance to leave his adolescent peer group, with its support-ive friendships and unrestricted dating.
  - ➤ Uncertainty about the loss of independence implied in accepting responsibility for a family with children.
  - ➤ Inability to loosen ties with his parents.

These ideas will be useful in constructing a plan of treatment.

DISSOCIATIVE

The phenomenon of dissociation, in which a person fails to integrate mem-ories, perceptions, a sense of identity, or consciousness of mental events, was originally associated with a group of conditions that in the late nine-teenth and early twentieth centuries were labeled "hysteria." Dissociation is linked with hypnosis, not only because, historically, hypnosis was com-monly used to treat hysteria, but also because the symptoms of dissocia-tive conditions so closely resemble a kind of self-hypnosis. Lumped into hysteria were, in today's nomenclature, conversion and somatic symp-tom disorders, borderline personality disorder, fugue states, dissocia-tive identity disorder, and PTSD. I have included all of these disparate diagnoses in the single category of "dissociative" because they all share a common etiology (dissociation) and thus contain common elements when constructing a formulation. Also included here would be patients whose central problems reflect difficulties in integrating their personal history with their current situation (Table 5–4).

In the last 75 years the United States has been involved in five armed conflicts that involved ground combat troops. These wars have generated so large a number of patients with PTSD that these cases represent the majority of dissociative illness. Smaller groups include survivors of nat-ural disasters, victims of crime (especially physical and sexual assault), and persons exposed to a variety of other experiences, such as automo-bile crashes, train wrecks, airplane crashes, and the like. Borderline per-sonality and dissociative identity disorders occur less frequently, and the other conditions in this category are uncommon.

CLINICAL EXAMPLE: A MAN STILL TRYING TO COPE WITH A LIFE-THREATENING EXPERIENCE

Dwayne is a 25-year-old former Marine lieutenant who survived an am-bush while leading his platoon on a dawn patrol in Helmand Province, Afghanistan. The ambush pinned them down in a shallow ditch. Auto-matic weapons fire and rocket-propelled grenades cut the air overhead,

---

TABLE 5–4. Dissociative category examples

Posttraumatic stress disorder

Dissociative identity disorder

Fugue states

Borderline personality disorder

Poor integration of past experience

Conversion disorder

Somatic symptom disorder

---

and mortar rounds shook the ground. Shrapnel blasted Dwayne's right leg. The headless torso of one of his Marines landed on top of him. Two years later he still has flashbacks, startle reactions to minor noises, and depression, and he has been unemployed since separation from the Corps on a medical discharge.

A striking fact about PTSD is how often it occurs in the absence of pre-existing psychiatric illness. Pierre Janet, a contemporary of Freud who originally defined the concept, believed that dissociation was a reparative function, an attempt at self-healing, rather than (as Freud thought) an illness reflecting unresolved childhood conflict. Whether someone develops posttraumatic symptoms almost always depends on the intensity and duration of the trauma, rather than on the presence of premorbid or disposing conditions. The longer a soldier is exposed to combat, for example, the more likely it is that he or she will develop PTSD. After twenty-four to thirty-six hours of continuous exposure, almost no one would survive without this problem.

A single, extremely intense life-threatening battle experience will also produce PTSD in a large percentage of soldiers, the way it did with Dwayne in the clinical example. We can assume he was free of psychiatric illness prior to the onset because he functioned at a high level as a Marine officer. He responded appropriately to the ambush, but his defenses were overwhelmed by his near death experience; the sights and sounds of battle, including burial under the body of one of his Marines; and a severe shrapnel wound. Absent the traumatic event, he would no doubt have continued to do well in his military role. In addition to our hypothesis that he functioned without psychiatric disability prior to the ambush, we can also hypothesize:

- His symptoms represent a failure to integrate the traumatic experience.

- Secondary problems—the loss of his military career, residual disability from his shrapnel wound, and his unemployment—contribute to his depression and his low level of function.

SITUATIONAL

Every one of us has a finite ability to cope with the stresses and disruptions of our daily lives. This coping ability usually allows us to function at a reasonable level in spite of the pressures of living. Sometimes, however, these pressures exceed our ability to deal with them, and at that point we develop stress-related symptoms like anxiety or a depressed mood. Some will turn to self-medication with alcohol or other drugs. Some will withdraw and lose the ability to function at their usual level. The stress may aggravate underlying pathologies that were not significant before but now become diagnosable disorders. Examples might include obsessional symptoms that were previously in the background or sexual problems previously well controlled. Sometimes stress aggravates personality traits and elevates them to the level of a personality disorder. If, after the passage of time or the onset of favorable developments in the environment, the level of stress declines again, these symptoms and symptomatic behaviors may disappear, allowing the individual to resume his or her prior level of satisfactory function. Sometimes, however, the damage caused by the disruption has altered patients' coping ability or their life circumstances so that they do not fully recover even when the cause of their difficulties is behind them.

Figure 5–3 illustrates the effect of stress on symptom development. In the boxes marked "maybe," symptoms might be intermittent: minor fluctuations in environmental stress levels, real or perceived, can cause symptoms to appear and disappear, on a day-to-day or on a less frequent basis. These variations may make recognition of this category more difficult. Part of the evaluation of patients with situational illness should include a determination of their previous coping ability. If you know their strengths and weaknesses, you can anticipate how well they will recover and what kinds of therapeutic interventions will be helpful.

An aspect of situational stress that may be underappreciated is that positive change is also stressful, and that events associated with good outcomes can be as difficult as those with bad results. These effects are seen in a scale that ranks events in terms of their "units of stress." The ranking resulted from a study of more than five thousand people that was set up to measure how stress affected the onset of physical illness.

	Coping Ability		
	Low	**Moderate**	**High**
Low Stress	Maybe	No	No
Moderate Stress	Yes	Maybe	No
High Stress	Yes	Yes	Maybe

FIGURE 5–3. Situational stress: will symptoms develop?

The study, by Holmes and Rahe,[7] showed that the more units of stress piled up, the greater the probability that the individual would become physically ill.

Table 5–5 illustrates the scale of life stress units. Death of a spouse was arbitrarily assigned 100 units, and the other events were graded in relation to it. Note that events such as marriage and retirement are high on the list. "Outstanding personal achievement" received a significant stress rating despite its positive value. About a third of the events are listed as "change," with the stress the same whether that change is for the better or the worse. Remember that the effects of a series of stressful events are cumulative: pregnancy, a job change, and a child leaving for college together create almost as much stress as the death of a spouse. What all this tells us is that a patient whose symptoms are stress related may be reacting to the accumulated effects of several changes, over time, not all of which appear to be harmful, or even significant, but whose combined impact is substantial.

CLINICAL EXAMPLE: A WORRIED MOTHER

Sheila, a 25-year-old married mother of two, was an active, outgoing wife and mother until her younger daughter, Linda, contracted meningitis shortly after her second birthday. Linda was in intensive care for

---

[7]Holmes TH, Rahe RH: "The Social Readjustment Rating Scale." *Journal of Psychosomatic Research* 11(2):213–218, 1967.

TABLE 5–5. Life stress units

Event	Life change units
Death of a spouse	100
Divorce	73
Marital separation	65
Imprisonment	63
Death of a close family member	63
Personal injury or illness	53
Marriage	50
Dismissal from work	47
Marital reconciliation	45
Retirement	45
Change in health of family member	44
Pregnancy	40
Sexual difficulties	39
Gain a new family member	39
Business readjustment	39
Change in financial state	38
Death of a close friend	37
Change to different line of work	36
Change in frequency of arguments	35
Major mortgage	32
Foreclosure of mortgage or loan	30
Change in responsibilities at work	29
Child leaving home	29
Trouble with in-laws	29
Outstanding personal achievement	28
Spouse starts or stops work	26
Beginning or end school	26
Change in living conditions	25
Revision of personal habits	24
Trouble with boss	23
Change in working hours or conditions	20
Change in residence	20
Change in schools	20
Change in recreation	19
Change in church activities	19
Change in social activities	18
Minor mortgage or loan	17
Change in sleeping habits	16
Change in number of family reunions	15
Change in eating habits	15
Vacation	13
Major holiday	12
Minor violation of law	11

Source.   Holmes and Rahe 1967.

three weeks before finally making an apparently good recovery. Sheila remained at the girl's bedside for the first ten days and hardly left the hospital until Linda was discharged. Sheila remains anxious, waking several times each night to check on her daughter, and is still losing weight ("I'm not hungry") and avoiding any separation from Linda during the day ("I still worry she'll relapse"). Her husband is losing patience with her, and her older daughter has become quiet and withdrawn.

In this example a single stressful event, "change in health of a family member" (44 life stress units), is enough to overwhelm the coping ability of this young mother. More ominous, however, is the persistence of symptoms after the problem is resolved. We might expect to find some underlying vulnerability in Sheila's background, or even guilt that she was not a good mother who could keep Linda safe, but we do not yet have sufficient history to explore either hypothesis. All we can say at this point is that Sheila appears to operate under the irrational (and somewhat narcissistic, if not grandiose) premise: "Unless I am vigilant and physically present to protect her, Linda will die."

TRANSACTIONAL

This category includes two types of patient presentations:

Type One: *Patients with interpersonal problems that result from dysfunctional relationships.* Conflicts between the patient and significant others will create tension and discord, such as between family members, spouses, and those with positions of power, like employers or supervisors. Although intrapsychic mechanisms undoubtedly contribute to the conflicts, a more effective therapy approach will center on the interactions between the patient and others, rather than the unresolved psychological problems that aggravate them.

Type Two: *Patients with personality trait problems that impact relationships.* Personality traits that are ego syntonic[8] will cause difficulties with other people. Personality disorders will show up here because these patients will not recognize their own stimulus value but instead will see only the results of those stimuli. They do not anticipate or recognize how their behavior impacts other people.

---

[8]*Ego syntonic* refers to those parts of one's personality that are acceptable and in keeping with one's self-image, including attitudes, ideas, impulses and behavior that others might consider problematic. For example, perfectionism may drive others crazy but seem perfectly reasonable to someone with an obsessional personality.

The old adage "Troublesome people are often people in trouble" reflects the external focus of this kind of patient. Therapy for patients with personality disorders may, of course, focus on the intrapsychic structures that are expressed in these behaviors. Psychoanalysis, for instance, will often target unresolved conflicts from the first six years of life as expressed through the transference. These efforts are typically long-term, and their success rate is not high. The transactional focus, with its effort to modify current behavior, may be more successful, especially with patients whose motivation and resources do not allow years of treatment.

An interesting model of interpersonal relationships was proposed by Eric Berne as part of what he called "transactional analysis."[9] He divided personality into three "ego states":

- The parent (either preaching or nurturing)
- The adult (objective, adaptable)
- The child (either oppositional or compliant)

The person-to-person exchanges among these ego states produce either complementary or crossed relationships. Complementary interactions run smoothly. For example, if one person criticizes another, acting as a critical parent, and the second person accepts the correction, acting as a compliant child, their transaction is mutually reinforcing. If the first person takes an adult position and the other a parental one, their crossed transaction creates conflict and dysphoria.

In Berne's theory, the problems caused by transactional dysfunction could become long-standing patterns of behavior that he called *scripts* and sometimes lead to recurring interpersonal schemes he called *games*. An example of a script is the repetitive efforts by the daughter of an alcoholic father to "rescue" a series of alcohol-addicted husbands. Her efforts inevitably fail, she despairs and divorces each of them, only to try again with a new relationship. A typical (and very familiar) game is "Why Don't You—Yes, But": the person playing the game presents a problem to a group but rejects each and every solution offered until every attempt at help has been denied and the group falls silent, thus demonstrating the gamer's superiority and control because no one can tell the player what to do.[10]

---

[9]Berne E: *Transactional Analysis in Psychotherapy*. New York, Grove Press, 1961.

[10]Berne's discussion of common games struck a responsive chord in the general public, and his book *Games People Play: The Psychology of Human Relationships* (New York, Grove Press, 1964) became a bestseller.

As an illustration (Figure 5–4), suppose you stopped your car to ask a pedestrian how to get to the Interstate. If the other person politely gave you directions, your adult-adult interaction would be complementary (*left diagram*). You are pleased to have the help, and the pedestrian is gratified to have been of assistance. If your request for help is met with a tirade of abuse ("Can't you see I'm busy? You should get yourself a GPS. You tourists are all the same..."), the interaction would be crossed (*right diagram*). Your adult request was answered with a critical parent response that would leave both of you upset and dissatisfied.

In individual psychotherapy, of course, only one party to the transactional problem is available. Fortunately, if your patient is able to modify his or her contribution to the interpersonal problem, the shift can cause the other person to alter the problem behavior in turn. This one-sided stimulus would change the outcome of the pathological interaction. In the crossed transaction for driving directions, for example, you could respond with a complementary stance as the compliant child ("You're right, I shouldn't bother you, but I'm hopelessly lost and you looked like someone who knew the area"). This response might elicit an adult reaction ("Okay, I'm sorry. It's been a bad day. Here's how you get there...") and restore the complementary balance. As an alternative, you could meet the critical parent with a crossed response in the form of your own critical parent ("What's wrong with you? Can't you answer a polite request and help someone who's lost?"). Perhaps that response would prompt the other person to tell you how to get to the interstate, or he could tell you where to go in other terms.

CLINICAL EXAMPLE: "FRIGID WOMAN" GAME

Theresa is a 25-year-old woman married for three years who reports increasing tension in the marriage over the issue of sex. She complains that her husband, Tom, has bad timing: whenever he wants to make love she is not ready and puts him off. She thinks he only wants sex, while she craves intimacy. Now he is calling her "frigid," and they are both angry and isolated. This pattern has been repeating, and worsening, over the last two years. When she notices him losing interest, she tries to flirt with him and excite him, but each time, when he finally responds, it is again at the wrong moment.

Berne described this transaction (in politically incorrect terminology: it *was* 1964) as the game "Frigid Woman," an unspoken collusion between the partners to avoid, or at least minimize, sexual intimacy. Further history may suggest reasons for Theresa's part in the game—for example, she may have had a seductive father whose flirtatious behavior both at-

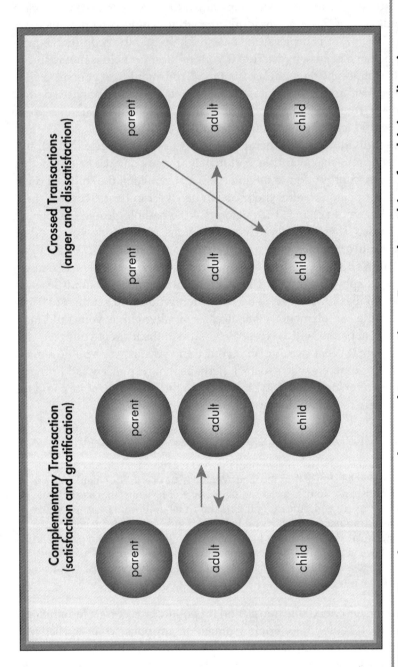

FIGURE 5–4. Complementary and crossed transactions. Example: asking for driving directions.

tracted and frightened her—but we do not necessarily need a dynamic explanation to treat her. Whatever her motives (and her husband's, because they are equal contributors to the problem), their *behavior* shows that they wish to avoid intimacy, even if they say the opposite. Since Tom is not involved in the therapy, we would explore this contradiction with Theresa under the hypothesis: you and Tom are struggling in your relationship *because* both of you want to avoid sexual intimacy.

EXISTENTIAL

We all face existential problems: the meaninglessness of our individual life, the inevitability of death, our isolation from others in an uncaring universe (Table 5–6). These philosophical and religious issues are always present, but in the ordinary course of life, not in the forefront of our thoughts.

When events or the natural flow of adult maturation brings any of these issues into focus, some of us manage to cope with them, perhaps with the help of social, cultural, or religious supports, but others cannot. We can function in spite of these disruptive ideas if, through denial, the use of social and cultural structures, or our own personal integrity, we are able to maintain an existential equilibrium between our defenses and these frightening realities. When patients whose equilibrium has failed consult us, we will be better able to help them if we recognize the problem and correctly understand it as an existential one, rather than focus on symptoms that derive from it, such as depression and anxiety.

TABLE 5–6. Existential concepts in psychotherapy

Existential concept	Issues in psychotherapy
Death	1. Perception of life's ending as stimulus to change in mental outlook
	2. Fundamental source of anxiety
Freedom	1. Responsibility for personal behavior
	2. Willingness to change behavior
Isolation	1. Impenetrable barrier between self and others
	2. Elemental cause of anxiety
Meaninglessness	1. Insignificance of one's individual life
	2. Personal significance in an indifferent universe

Source. Adapted from Yalom ID: *Existential Psychotherapy*. New York, Basic Books, 1980.

CLINICAL EXAMPLE: THE REALITY OF DEATH

Esther, a 45-year-old single woman, abruptly resigned her teaching position at a local college after her older brother, Eddie, died suddenly from a ruptured cerebral aneurysm. She remained alone in her one-bedroom apartment and only left to buy food and to walk late at night when she could not sleep. Her friends became worried when she did not answer her telephone or come to the door, and they called the police. Although she insisted she was all right, she was transported to the emergency room and seen by a psychiatrist. In the consultation she reported that Eddie had been her hero and that since his death she recognized that striving was pointless. "Life is shit," she said, "and then you die."

Esther appears to have been functioning normally, busy with her life and her career, until her brother's sudden and unexpected death. Eddie was only a few years older, and his death has broken through the "normal" feeling of immortality that supports most people in early to middle adulthood. Esther now realizes she is vulnerable and her lifespan is unknown. She thinks:

- Could I have an aneurysm too?
- What's the point of going to work if it all could end at any time?
- Does my life mean anything?

It is the impact of these doubts, on top of her grief and sense of loss after Eddie's death, that has disrupted her life and created feelings of hopelessness and despair. At this point, we do not have sufficient history to explain why Esther is especially vulnerable to this loss, but we may be able to help her without this knowledge. Our hypothesis is that Esther's paralysis and withdrawal occurred *because* her brother's death destabilized her existential equilibrium.

PSYCHODYNAMIC

The central idea that defines this category is that desires, beliefs, events, attitudes, and emotions encountered or generated earlier in life, sometimes before the acquisition of language, shape our current behavior. This historical approach postulates that these dynamics[11] are constantly at

---

[11]The word *dynamic* here means a psychological force that creates intrapsychic change.

work, often out of consciousness, to determine—indeed, to overdetermine[12]—what we think, feel, and do in the present. Originally a concept on which Sigmund Freud based his psychoanalytic theory, the idea has now stimulated many methodologies, not only those derived directly from Freud but also many independent therapies.

CLINICAL EXAMPLE: A PROBLEM OF SUCCESS

Phillip, a 35-year-old graduate of Harvard Business School, was recently promoted to vice-president of his company. As he entered his new office (bigger and better furnished), he became short of breath, light-headed, and weak. When he complained of chest pain, he was transported to the emergency room, but a workup found no cardiac disease, and he was told he had had an anxiety attack. He is the first in his family to go to college. His father, who died a year earlier, worked construction. He had been thinking of his father just before his panic attack. He feels guilty at his "good fortune" of succeeding so far beyond what anyone in his family ever did. He cannot believe he deserved his rapid promotion and wonders when he will be "found out."

Trying to understand the psychodynamic basis for Phillip's panic attack with only this snippet of his history is mere guesswork. Does entering his new office, the physical manifestation of his success, mean

- His new social and economic status will isolate him from his family?
- He fears retaliation from the (introjected[13]) father he has now outshone?
- He feels unconscious guilt over his father's death?
- He has betrayed his father and rejected him as a model?

We do not know whether one or more of these ideas caused the panic, and we cannot know without more data about his childhood relationships with both parents, as well as his developmental history, his other interpersonal relationships, and a lot more. As a guess we can hypothesize that his reaction is likely related to unresolved oedipal issues, perhaps aggravated by his father's recent death.

---

[12]*Overdetermination*: a single effect is the result of multiple causes, even though any one of them alone might be sufficient.

[13]An *introjected object* is an internalized, mental representation that may be a distorted version of an actual person or idea and survives unchanged within the psyche, where it is treated emotionally as real.

Choosing the Right Category

Sometimes the assignment to one of these seven categories is an easy decision. The patient's history and clinical presentation fit the criteria, and no other category seems appropriate. When the choice is not clear, it can be facilitated by a "process of elimination." You can go down the list and determine which ones do not match:

- If no organic or physiological condition is present, then it is *not* biological.
- If the patient does not confront a stage of life transition, then it is *not* developmental.
- If there is no history of trauma or abuse and no memory distortions, then it is *not* dissociative.
- If the patient's symptoms have not developed in response to immediate, increased life stresses, then it is *not* situational.
- If the problem is not primarily interpersonal, then it is *not* transactional.
- If the patient does not confront an existential crisis (death, responsibility, isolation, lack of meaning), then it is *not* existential.
- If the patient's current dilemma is not historically related to earlier unresolved conflict, then it is *not* psychodynamic.

At times, however, the patient's history may not fit cleanly into only one of the categories. Instead, two or three categories may overlap. For example:

- Some aspects are stress-related and some are interpersonal.
- Some features will be developmental and some psychodynamic.
- A patient with major depression may report that life seems meaningless.
- A person with a history of trauma may confront current, unusual stressors.

In these mixed cases, the best solution is to choose the category that is the most

- Recent.
- Significant.
- Important to the patient.

In addition to these criteria, choose a category based on which one will yield the most useful set of treatment goals. Other, less important issues can be addressed at a later point or may become more significant as therapy progresses, and the treatment plan can be revised accordingly.

What the choice of a single category tries to accomplish is not absolute certainty (a rare commodity anyway) but a reasonable starting point, a frame of reference within which the clinical data can be organized into a useful explanation of the patient's history.

The formulation is a tool, an organizational step to make sense of the patient's presentation. You can use the formulation at first for your own clarification of the important treatment objectives and later to explain these goals to your patient.

Final Thoughts

An appreciation of the importance of a formulation and its role in organizing therapy is a key element in an effective therapy. If you understand why your patient has his or her presenting problems—where they came from and what role they play—you can convert a complex history into a set of useful constructs. Your understanding of the central issues that impact your patient will allow you to plan and conduct a successful therapy. The challenge in this important step has always been the significant difficulty posed by the required use of the inductive process. By making that step a deductive exercise, as clinically familiar as deciding on a diagnosis, that hurdle may be largely overcome. Cause-and-effect decisions suggest themselves more easily when confronted within the limited framework each category provides. Cause-and-effect ideas lead readily to therapy goals and the development of a workable treatment plan. These next steps are discussed in the following chapter.

Key Points

- Although often neglected, the formulation is a critical element of planning treatment for a successful therapy.

- A complete formulation will include 1) a brief clinical description, 2) relevant history with cause-and-effect hypotheses, and 3) a summary.

- The challenge of inductive reasoning creates a barrier to formulation.

- The substitution of an initial deductive step, similar to making a diagnosis, can lessen the formulation challenge.

- Seven inclusive categories—biological, developmental, dissociative, situational, transactional, existential, and psychodynamic—are offered to facilitate this step.

- When a patient's history falls into more than one category, choose the one most recent, significant, and important to the patient.

CHAPTER SIX

What Is a Treatment Plan?

It is a bad plan that admits of no modification.

Publilius Syrus, Maxim 469

You've got to be very careful if you don't know where you are going, because you might not get there.

Yogi Berra

Introduction

You met your new patient, established a working relationship, and explored the chief complaint, the present illness, and as much of the history as you could cover in the initial interview. You marshaled the data to form one or more hypotheses. You put together a reasonable formulation that explains the why and the how of the patient's problems. Now you can take the result of all this work and organize it into a roadmap of the therapy to come. What will be the treatment outcome and how will that be accomplished?

Even though you (and the patient) are eager to get started, this final task necessarily imposes a certain amount of restraint. Not only must you pause to complete the mental exercise involved, you must also explain your ideas to the patient and negotiate an agreement on the work you propose. The agreement should be overt: to assume the patient knows what you have in mind and agrees with it and is ready to engage in the therapy process is to invite failure.

- What the patient wants (as you have elicited in the interview) and what you think should happen must be congruent.
- Agreement on the process invites collaboration and reduces resistance.
- If your formulation is accurate, given your current knowledge, it can only help the patient to hear what it is.

183

Definition

A *treatment plan*, in its simplest form, is a statement of

- The result you anticipate from a period of therapy.
- The intermediate objectives that will bring about that result.
- The process by which you and the patient together will work to achieve it.

To construct a treatment plan, you will need four steps:

1. *Decide on the desired outcome.* This decision is the required initial step. What is the aim of your treatment? If it succeeds, how will the patient be better off?
2. *Choose the treatment goal(s).* Unless the therapy has a designated aim, you have no basis for the second step, the choice of treatment goals. What specific accomplishments will achieve the desired outcome?
3. *Determine the methodology.* Once you have decided on the objectives, you can pick the methodology you will use to reach them. What is the most effective therapy approach for each of the goals?
4. *Pick the techniques.* Unless you know which therapy you need to reach each goal, you cannot choose the techniques the process will require.

Stated in these simple terms it may seem that the value of these decisions is obvious. Alas, it is not. Treatment planning has its detractors as well as its adherents.

Opposing Camps

The idea that psychotherapy should follow a plan—and, indeed, whether planned therapy is even possible—divides therapists into two apparently irreconcilable camps. In one camp are those who favor planning. They argue that it is

- Possible to select the best outcome suggested by the initial evaluation.
- More efficient to tailor the therapy work toward specific treatment objectives.
- More effective to follow a plan.

In the other camp, those who oppose planning believe that

- Planning is too restrictive and limits progress.
- Therapy issues arise from associations and interventions that cannot be predicted.
- It is impossible to foresee a therapy outcome in advance.

To some extent, which camp you are in depends on what kind of therapy you mean to do. Those who favor a structured therapy—a behavioral treatment, for instance —will want a clear treatment plan. Proponents of unstructured therapy—an existential treatment, perhaps—will reject the idea of a plan.

- In cognitive-behavioral therapy (CBT), the patient is directed to deal with specific subjects.
- In psychoanalytic work, the patient's undirected associations lead the therapy in unplanned and unanticipated directions.

Both therapies expect improvement to result from these contradictory methodological approaches. And even the unstructured therapy proponent has some kind of plan. For example, a psychoanalyst-in-training once told me that the analyst should not say anything to the patient for the first year of analysis, presumably because the analyst is waiting for the right kind of material to emerge. "Don't speak for a year" is a plan, no matter how extreme or whatever its wisdom.

The underlying question is: do we want psychotherapy to have a definable benefit?

- In both psychoanalysis and CBT, patients sometimes (or even often) return for second or third or fourth courses of treatment. This pattern suggests that the outcomes have been incomplete, transitory, or illusory.
- Sometimes the period of treatment has no recognizable endpoint. The patient either drifts away or drops out, but in either case terminates therapy without your agreement.
- Some patients simply continue to attend indefinitely, with no discernible further improvement. They may continue for the therapeutic alliance alone, perhaps with the camouflage of repetition or reinforcement of earlier therapy interventions, but with no new progress.

- Among the general public, and in the view of some mental health practitioners, this "interminable" treatment is evidence against the idea that psychotherapy really works.
- Interminable treatment suggests that therapy is not a cure but a lifestyle. The filmmaker Woody Allen was reportedly in psychoanalysis for 37 years—*37 years!*—but in spite of all of this treatment still suffers from agoraphobia and claustrophobia. In today's cost-conscious, third-party environment, never-ending therapy becomes increasingly harder to justify.

Perhaps the disagreement about treatment plans is not as intransigent as it appears from the discussion above. After all, both sides must agree that

- Therapy should *have* an outcome, or else why undertake such a difficult and expensive effort?
- A defined process is required, or else what distinguishes therapy from an ordinary conversation?
- Therapy requires the combined efforts of you and the patient to reach the anticipated result using the required process, or else why does the patient need you? (Table 6–1)

TABLE 6–1. Therapy versus "conversation"

Dyadic therapy	Dyadic conversation
Defined outcome	Open-ended
Relationship plus defined process	Relationship only
Therapist necessary	No professional role
Training required	No training needed

On closer inspection, then, it appears that the dispute is over the "how" and the "why" rather than the "what." It is a disagreement over the pathway to be followed rather than the destination of the journey, even if that destination might be described in different terms, depending on the language of the journey's guide. In other words, the two sides have differing beliefs about how therapy should work and why it helps patients improve. They apparently agree on the idea that *therapy should achieve a result*, an outcome, from the application of the particular treatment they support.

If the two viewpoints agree on the desirability of an outcome, however, they may still disagree that it requires a plan to get there. The alternative is a belief that the process will, if followed correctly, inevitably reach the optimal outcome, although the path it may follow is unpredictable. Underlying this belief are the following principles:

- The therapist is passive and makes no effort to influence the direction the therapy takes.
- The patient determines the entire course of therapy.
- The therapist follows the patient's progress and occasionally helps or facilitates the patient's efforts.

Therapists who find this stance congenial, however, may be unaware of their own influence, and, arguably, they have abdicated their fundamental responsibility as a healing force.

At its core, the disagreement also rests on the underlying assumption that the therapist can, and should, offer only one "process." In the above dichotomy, a therapist is restricted to either psychodynamic psychotherapy or CBT, but not both. One is to be considered effective and the other is not. A great deal of paper and much ink (not to mention, bytes and pixels) have been utilized to debate this question without much progress to resolve it.

Suppose, however, that you can choose either process—either a psychodynamic approach or a cognitive one—depending on your judgment as to which would be more effective in dealing with a particular patient's problems. There is no credible evidence that says one particular therapy is better than all the others, although there is some evidence, both anecdotal and researched, that one therapy might be better than another for a specific type of problem. If different methodologies can be used to help a patient recover, perhaps the disagreement over planning will be less intense. Different therapies can even be used within a single course of treatment, each one directed at a problem for which it is more effective. In that circumstance, it would seem that the opposing camps might be united, or at least agree to a truce.

This chapter approaches the issue with three assumptions:

1. Psychotherapy does work.
2. Some therapies work better than others *in particular cases.*
3. A defined outcome is necessary for it to succeed.

These ideas place me firmly in the first camp—that planning is both possible and desirable—but my argument will not, I suspect, alter the belief systems of those in the opposing camp.

The Prototype Plan

I have advocated a four-level plan[1] that is illustrated in Figure 6–1.

1. *Aim.* At the top level, the desired outcome, the *aim,* should be the overall desired result of a course of treatment. Each period of treatment can have only one aim. It should
   a. Resolve the distress that brought the patient to you.
   b. Restore the patient to at least the previous level of function, and perhaps to even a higher level.
   c. Allow the patient to make further progress and growth and development.
2. *Goals.* On the second level, the aim can be realized with the completion of one or more (usually two to four) *goals.* Each of these objectives addresses a component of the effort needed to reach the aim.
3. *Strategy.* The third level stipulates the choice of methods. To achieve each goal will require a particular *strategy,* the methodology best suited for the patient and for the expected result. Sometimes a single treatment modality will suffice for all the goals, or one modality will be directed toward two of the goals but not all of them.
4. *Tactics.* The final level designates the tools needed for the specified strategies. Each strategy has its own set of techniques, or *tactics,* that are required for its successful application.

Figure 6–2 shows how a more complex treatment plan might be diagrammed.

Top Down Versus Bottom Up

Planning decisions should follow a logical sequence. You must have an aim before you can choose the goals needed to achieve it. Knowledge of the goals will allow you to make decisions about which are the best strategies for each. The choice of a strategy predicts which techniques you will need. This sequence outlines a top-down approach.

The opposite approach is, of course, the bottom-up. If you have decided you must immediately tackle each problem as soon as it appears,

---

[1]Makover RB: *Treatment Planning for Psychotherapists,* 3rd Edition. Arlington, VA, American Psychiatric Association Publishing, 2016.

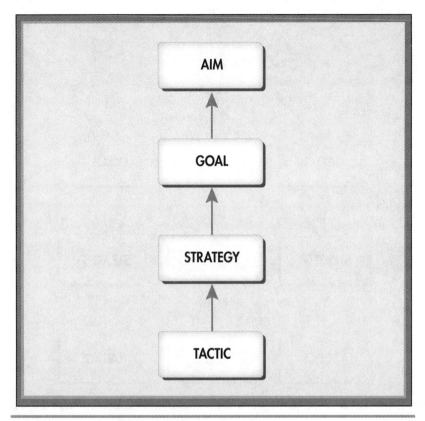

FIGURE 6-1. **Basic treatment plan.**

your focus will shift from the treatment outcome, the long-term view, to a short-term, troubleshooting effort. In the worst case, you will use a technique without an idea of its overall purpose.

Bottom-up decisions highlight two planning fallacies:

- The *strategic fallacy* is the belief that only a single treatment methodology is valid. When it is applied to the strategy level of the plan, the result is to limit the treatment possibilities. If, for example, the therapist is committed to a cognitive-behavioral strategy and chooses that method before deciding on the goals or the aim of the therapy, then the goals are reduced to a problem list. A concrete list does not capture the crux of the patient's problem and may miss important aspects of it. For example, a patient may present with phobic symptoms, and if you simply catalog the specific stimuli and environments that activate the avoidance as preparation for a behavioral intervention,

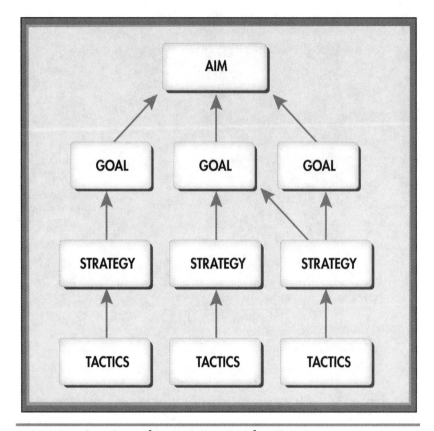

FIGURE 6–2. Complex treatment plan.

you can miss the context of the dependency and marital problems in which the avoidance occurs. If you recall the case vignette from Chapter Two,[2] Elizabeth's fear of driving over the Mianus River Bridge aggravated her dependent personality traits, and when she overcame the phobia, these traits became less of a problem too.

- The *technical fallacy* is a reliance on a particular set of procedural interventions without an appreciation for their relevance to the problem at hand. Applying a technique that is not part of a coordinated and coherent strategy can misdirect the therapist's efforts away from a major problem toward a minor one for which a technique seems warranted. In Chapter One,[3] we saw that Norman offered Lisa relaxation

---

[2]See pages 42–46.
[3]See page 18.

training before he knew the extent of her developmental and marital problems. To paraphrase the old adage: if your favorite tool is a wrench, you will only look for nuts. The bottom-up therapist treats symptoms, some or all of which may be tangential, while the focus on the patient's major problems is lost.

Planning Foundations

Planning decisions are based on the information and ideas generated from the initial evaluation.

- You combine the history and the hypotheses from the interview into a formulation.
- Your formulation identifies the major issues confronting the patient, and it generates cause-and-effect conclusions about how these problems came about.
- These conclusions identify the most desirable outcome, the therapy's aim.
- A decision as to the aim of the therapy leads you naturally into a determination of which goals will lead to an effective and helpful outcome.

Planning must, in other words, proceed from the general to the particular:

- From the abstract idea embodied in the aim to the more specific decisions about the goals that must be accomplished to reach it.
- From the more general concept of those overall objectives to conclusions about what particular methodology will best allow the patient to attain them.
- From the choice of a methodology to the concrete decisions about particular techniques that will be effective in carrying it out.

All of these planning decisions are deductive in nature (deduction follows a path from the general to the particular), and, as we saw earlier, deduction is easier than inductive reasoning.

In hierarchical systems, knowledge about one level will not tell us about the levels above and below it.

- Knowing about a liver cell will not explain how the liver functions.
- Knowing about a group will not predict the behavior of its individual members.

It is important to understand each level of the plan, the characteristics of the aim, of each goal, and of the strategies selected. If you identify a single treatment goal, without the concept of an overall result that is supplied by the aim, your decision does not lead to other important goals or an idea about the aim of the therapy as a whole. If you choose a particular type of psychotherapy and decide to use it for a patient before you know what the patient's problems require, you foreclose any other possible methods of treatment, some of which could be more effective and more likely to succeed with that patient and with those problems.

A therapy that begins with incorrect or partially correct decisions about what must be done is more likely to fail. It will deteriorate into unfocused efforts or result in a therapeutic impasse in which progress ceases and no further work can be accomplished.

Examples of Planning

To see how a formulation can translate into a treatment plan, we can re-examine the clinical vignettes from the seven categories described in the previous chapter. Those brief case histories were used to illustrate each category and were not complete formulations because they did not include causation hypotheses or summaries. In each of the following examples, I have had to include certain hypotheses or assumptions that were not present in those very short descriptions in order to complete the formulation and to represent the process of planning in a more useful way. In an actual evaluation I would explore these hypotheses carefully as I sought additional data about the history and the current illness. I might also test these hypotheses with trial interpretations or other probative interventions.

BIOLOGICAL CATEGORY

> David is a 25-year-old single male graduate student who presents with a three-month history of depressed mood, insomnia, anorexia, and suicidal ideation without a plan. The diagnosis is major depressive disorder. The onset occurred after his fiancée broke their engagement. A previous romantic breakup when he was 17 was followed by a similar, though milder, episode that resolved without treatment. His father died when he was 11. His mother and maternal grandmother have had recurrent depressions. In summary, this 25-year-old man has a history of recurrent depression precipitated by loss of a close relationship in the context of early loss of his father and a family predisposition to depressive illness.

Case Formulation

This 25-year-old man has a three-month history of major depression precipitated by his broken engagement, with a prior episode also linked to a romantic breakup. He is susceptible to recurrent depression *because of* a positive family history. He is sensitive to these losses *because of* his father's death when he was 11. His vulnerability means he is at risk for future recurrences.

Treatment Plan

The Aim

My treatment plan must start with a decision about what result my therapy should accomplish. In this case, presented with clear evidence of depression, I can aim for its reversal. The opposite of depression could be "remission" or "recovery," but both these terms are nonspecific. More specific would be a result that brings David's depressed mood back to a normal mood level, the term for which is *euthymia*, a more accurate designation.

Goals

My next decision is, "What must happen for David to become euthymic?"

- Obviously, one of my goals must be to reverse the biological process that led to his depression. Since I cannot measure David's brain chemistry directly, I can state this goal as alleviate the depressive symptoms (i.e., depressed mood, insomnia, anorexia, and suicidal ideation).
- Another aspect of the depression is an alteration of cognition, marked by hopelessness, helplessness, and defeated ideation, perhaps focused on his negative beliefs about personal loss ("People leave me because I'm bad."). My second goal would be to revise this pattern of thought.
- Finally, because David has a prior history of depression, I want to help him avoid relapse after his recovery and minimize his vulnerability for future episodes. This third goal can be stated as "prevent recurrences."

To summarize, the three goals I have derived from my aim of euthymia are 1) alleviate depressive symptoms, 2) reverse depressive cognition, and 3) prevent recurrences.

Strategies and Tactics

My next question has to be, "How can I help David achieve these goals?"

- My "biological" diagnosis suggests I need a biological treatment to combat his depressed mood and its attendant symptoms. This strategy could be psychopharmacology. Notice that the answer is not a particular medication. That decision would be a tactic or technical decision and not a strategy in itself. At the tactical level, under the heading of psychopharmacology, I could list "an SSRI antidepressant" or I could be more specific and choose, for instance, fluoxetine as the antidepressant.
- The medication might also help David's depressive ideation, but a more specific strategy would be cognitive therapy. In fact, I could choose cognitive therapy instead of medication and have one strategy for both goals, or even all three goals. While medication alone and cognitive therapy alone are both effective treatments for depression, the two together can be more effective than either used by itself. If David declined medication, however, I could feel equally optimistic with only the cognitive therapy option.
- For my third goal, preventing recurrence, I could continue the cognitive therapy for "booster" visits, have David continue to take maintenance medication, and add education and direct reinforcement.

All of these decisions are shown in the planning diagram in Figure 6–3.

DEVELOPMENTAL CATEGORY

> Dennis is a 25-year-old lawyer who has doubts about his upcoming wedding to a woman he has known for five years. He wants to break the engagement, but a friend convinced him to see a therapist before making his decision. He is afraid to limit himself to just one relationship ("I'm too young to get married; how do I know she's the right one?"), he does not want to have a child and start a family ("I'm not ready for that kind of responsibility"), and he worries that it will impact his bond with his parents ("She's not as close to them as I'd like"). These anxieties have resulted in insomnia, a weight loss of twelve pounds, and increasing irritability with his fiancée. He resents her enthusiasm about the wedding plans. He hesitates to break the engagement, however, because he still loves her.

Case Formulation

This 25-year-old man presents with worries about his pending marriage that lead him to doubt his decision. His doubts reflect his difficulty with the transition from a bachelorhood rooted in his family of origin to the

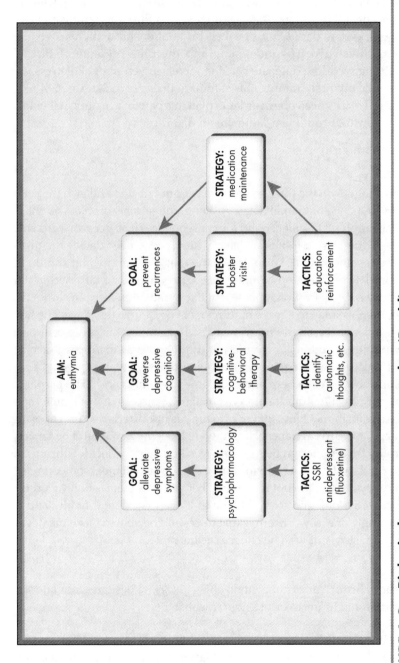

FIGURE 6–3. Biological category treatment plan (David).

responsibilities and limitations implied by marriage. He is anxious, in part, *because* marriage would mean giving up his peer group and his present lifestyle and taking on more responsibility (becoming a parent himself), and, in part, *because* he feels his relationship with his own parents is threatened. His indecision, and the time pressure of the approaching wedding date, are causing increasing emotional distress.

Unlike my first example, this summary does not include a DSM-5 diagnosis. I do not need one in order to plan this patient's treatment. For billing purposes, I could use "adjustment disorder."

Treatment Plan

The Aim

Dennis falters on the threshold of a maturational step and is in the early stages of a developmental delay. Although he sees his problem as one of indecision about his fiancée and the consequences if he goes forward with the wedding, larger issues are clearly involved. Once I decide the problem is developmental, I also determine that the therapy aim should be to complete the developmental process. A patient who falls within this category is, by definition, unable to make a transition from an earlier developmental stage to a more mature one. For Dennis this means he hesitates to leave the family he grew up in, to abandon his adolescent peer group and its "dating" activities, and to choose a single partner with whom he can begin a new family. Given this stalemate, the aim of my therapy should be to help him overcome his doubts and to be prepared to take the next maturational step. For short, I can call this outcome "successful transition." Note that my therapy is not directed at his choosing to marry his current fiancée. If that were true, my aim would be "marry Dorothy." Even though he says he loves her, he may decide, during the therapy, that she is not right for him. Perhaps he will meet someone else, or already has but has not mentioned her yet. Whether to marry Dorothy is a separate decision from the one to leave his original family and to form a new one. My concern is that he should be able to make the developmental step, not who he chooses as his mate.

Goals

My brief history does not contain clues to *why* he hesitates, but later exploration might uncover possible reasons:

- Although he loves her, Dorothy might not offer him a strong enough bond to justify letting go of the relationships he now has with family and peers.

- Unresolved problems with his parents may undermine his confidence in his ability to separate from them.
- Doubts about his parenting abilities may make him anxious about having children; for example, because of his increased irritability, he may think he is too short-tempered and might hurt his child in a fit of anger.

Future sessions with him will provide more information about his history that will perhaps require me to reformulate his case. For now, the goals I might set would be based on his stated reservations:

1. I'm too young to get married.
2. How do I know she's the right one?
3. I'm not ready for the responsibility of raising children.
4. I won't see as much of my parents.

These concerns might lead to the following goals:

1. Resolve doubts about his readiness to be married.
2. Overcome fears of parental responsibility.
3. Establish greater emotional distance from his family.

Strategies and Tactics

A useful strategy to deal with all three of these "intellectual" questions might be CBT. Although other methods could also work, Dennis is under some time pressure because of his approaching wedding date. Psychodynamic therapy could involve a broadly based investigation of this developmental step, but a more directive strategy like cognitive therapy would be a more efficient intervention to help him decide whether to proceed with the ceremony, call off the engagement, or perhaps delay the wedding.

These ideas are contained in the Figure 6–4 planning diagram.

DISSOCIATIVE CATEGORY

Dwayne is a 25-year-old former Marine lieutenant who survived an ambush while leading his platoon on a dawn patrol in Helmand Province, Afghanistan. The ambush pinned them down in a shallow ditch. Automatic weapons fire and rocket-propelled grenades cut the air overhead and mortar rounds shook the ground. Shrapnel blasted Dwayne's right leg. The headless torso of one of his Marines landed on top of him. Two years later he still has flashbacks, startle reactions to minor noises, and depression, and he has been unemployed since separation from the Corps on a medical discharge.

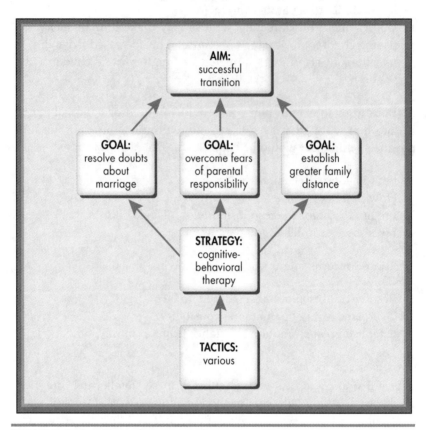

FIGURE 6–4. **Developmental category treatment plan (Dennis).**

Case Formulation

This 25-year-old man presents with posttraumatic stress disorder (PTSD) after a life-threatening combat incident. Dwayne has no known vulnerability *because* he functioned normally prior to the incident. He is disabled *because* he cannot integrate the battlefield event and deal with his response to it. These residual symptoms of a life-threatening experience prevent him from having a normal civilian life.

Treatment Plan

The Aim

With this young Marine I am dealing with the effects of a single traumatic event that resulted in a marked decrease in his level of function.

Prior to the ambush he was an officer commanding a platoon. He had a successful college career and would have gone on either to a full military career or private sector employment. My best outcome would be to return him to his pretrauma level of function, and I can translate this result into an aim, "resume prior function."

Goals, Strategies, and Tactics

In dissociative disorders, where an experience or even a part of the personality has become isolated from the rest, recovery often involves reintegrating the dissociative elements to restore the integrity of the patient's mental function. I want him to integrate the traumatic experience and to do so he needs to

1. Decrease the effect of the remembered experience. (My strategy could be some form of exposure therapy, and I could consider using hypnosis.)
2. Increase his ability to cope with the effects of the trauma. (My efforts might include relaxation training, mindfulness, role-playing, and the like.)
3. Replace negative perceptions with more positive ideas. (Cognitive therapy would be a good approach for this goal.)
4. Gain relief, at least temporarily, for the dysphoria and anxiety. (Medication could help control those emotions.)

This plan is outlined in Figure 6–5.

SITUATIONAL CATEGORY

> Sheila, a 25-year-old married mother of two, was an active, outgoing wife and mother until her younger daughter, Linda, contracted meningitis shortly after her second birthday. Linda was in intensive care for three weeks before finally making an apparently good recovery. Sheila remained at the girl's bedside for the first ten days and hardly left the hospital until Linda was discharged. Sheila remains anxious, waking several times each night to check on her daughter, and is still losing weight ("I'm not hungry") and avoiding any separation from Linda during the day ("I still worry she'll relapse"). Her husband is losing patience with her, and her older daughter has become quiet and withdrawn.

Case Formulation

This 25-year-old woman presents with an adjustment disorder with anxious mood precipitated by her daughter's hospitalization with menin-

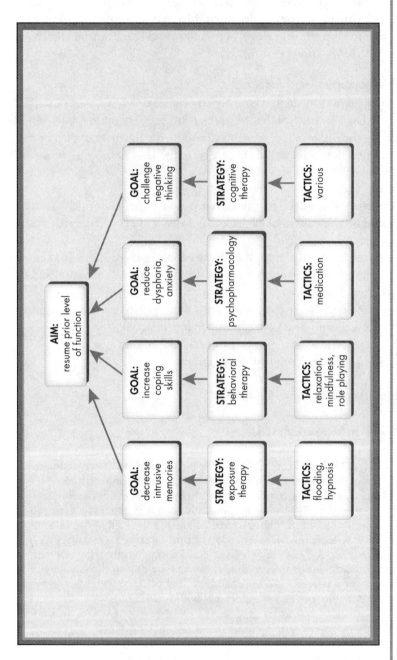

FIGURE 6–5. Dissociative category treatment plan (Dwayne).

gitis. She continues to treat her daughter as a critically ill patient *because* of a false belief that her child, who is now well, remains in danger. Her inability to accept the child's recovery may be *because* she feels guilty about her getting sick. Her anxious and perhaps guilty behavior is having a negative impact on her family.

Treatment Plan

The Aim
Once again my aim is for the patient to resume her previous, normal level of function.

Goals, Strategies, and Tactics
In the absence of further clinical information, and for the purpose of this exercise, I can speculate (on the basis of some common dynamic ideas) that Sheila's recovery is blocked by an irrational guilt that she was somehow responsible for her daughter's life-threatening illness. As punishment she is not eating, an overdetermined response because it

- Deprives her of the enjoyment of eating, and therefore represents a deserved punishment.
- Mimics Linda's inability to eat during her illness and may indicate she has identified with her child.
- Symbolically threatens her with death from starvation, or retribution for her "sin."

At the same time her obsessive checking behavior that keeps her at Linda's side is an attempt to suppress the anxiety that was legitimately generated by Linda's severe illness but now continues even though the child is well. What was appropriate in the hospital persists as an unwanted symptom. The goal of relief from undeserved guilt can be treated with psychodynamic psychotherapy. Exposure and response prevention, a behavioral approach, can be used for the checking behavior. This treatment plan is diagrammed in Figure 6–6.

TRANSACTIONAL CATEGORY

Theresa is a 25-year-old woman married for three years who reports increasing tension in the marriage over the issue of sex. She complains that her husband, Tom, has bad timing: whenever he wants to make love she is not ready and puts him off. She thinks he only wants sex while she craves intimacy. Now he is calling her "frigid," and they are both angry and isolated. This pattern has been repeated, and has worsened, over the

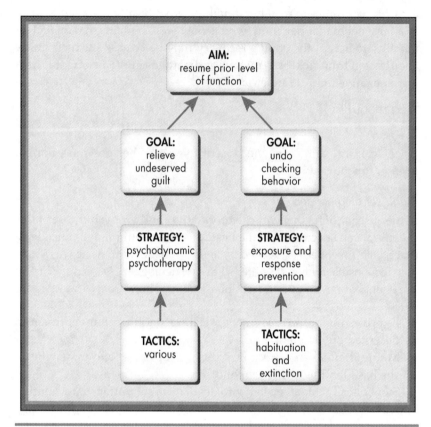

FIGURE 6–6.   Situational category treatment plan (Sheila).

last two years. When she notices Tom losing interest she tries to flirt with
him and excite him, but each time, when he finally responds, it is again
at the wrong moment.

Case Formulation

This 25-year-old woman presents with a deteriorating marital relationship
as a result of increasing sexual conflict. Formal diagnosis is deferred.
Their struggle over sexual intimacy remains unresolved *because* neither
can gain control over this aspect of their relationship, and *because* avoiding sex may serve their mutual needs. The repetitive interaction has the
characteristics of a "game" *because* the ostensible subject—when and
whether to make love—conceals both a deeper disagreement over which
will be the dominant partner and a covert agreement to avoid intimacy.
Although they have only been married for three years, this escalating
battle threatens to dissolve the marriage.

This couple's predicament is transactional because it represents a shared effort to avoid making love as well as a power struggle between the two partners. When either of them gains the upper hand (by controlling sexual activity), both are losers. Tom also, we assume, "wins" the game of sexual avoidance when he turns down her flirtatious advances, meaning he is in charge, but probably feels spurned and alone. Theresa rejects his advances, leaving her in charge, but feels misunderstood, neglected, and unloved. Theresa too "wins" because she is avoiding intimacy as well. The stability of this game reflects the way it gratifies the needs of both partners, who secretly, perhaps unconsciously, agree on the restriction of their sexual behavior.

Treatment Plan

The Aim

If I assume this couple's marriage is otherwise satisfactory, as it seems to be from the available information, the aim can be to improve their sexual relationship. As therapy proceeds, of course, I might uncover other significant problems. If so, I would reformulate the case and modify the treatment plan.

Goals

Couple's therapy might be an effective approach, but since only one partner is available, Theresa must realize she can only change Tom's behavior by changing her own. In other words, if she alters the pattern of their transactions, it will encourage Tom to alter his. Three goals that will help her toward a more satisfactory sexual relationship would be

1. Open better communication links with Tom.
2. Change the power struggle to mutual power sharing.
3. Expand their sexual repertoire to include affectionate, mutually acceptable activities.

Strategies and Tactics

A useful strategy for Theresa's therapy would be transactional analysis. That interpersonal model could demonstrate to her the gamesmanship and crossed transactions inherent in the couple's script and would provide a framework for her to understand, and then alter, the self-defeating behavior they have both adopted.

Contrast this approach with a psychodynamic therapy that would explore Theresa's problems with intimacy, looking for childhood issues that would explain it, or a cognitive approach that would try to identify a core belief, such as "If I give in to Tom, I'll lose control and be helpless" or "Being physically intimate means I'll lose my identity as an independent person." Neither methodology would focus the therapy on the marriage itself, an oversight that could allow the marital problems to escalate and even end in divorce.

These ideas are reflected in the treatment plan in Figure 6–7.

EXISTENTIAL CATEGORY

> Esther, a 45-year-old single woman, abruptly resigned her teaching position at a local college after her older brother, Eddie, died suddenly from a ruptured cerebral aneurysm. She remained alone in her one-bedroom apartment and only left to buy food and to walk late at night when she could not sleep. Her friends became worried when she did not answer her telephone or come to the door, and they called the police. Although she insisted she was all right, she was transported to the emergency room and seen by a psychiatrist. In the consultation she reported that Eddie had been her hero, and that since his death she recognized that striving was pointless. "Life is shit," she quoted, "and then you die."

Case Formulation

This 45-year-old woman has retreated into isolation and self-neglect after the sudden death of her brother. The diagnosis is adjustment disorder with mixed disturbance of emotions and conduct. Most of the time we all exist in a state of denial about our mortality: yes, we are going to die, but not now and not for a long time. When an event breaks through this curtain of denial and confronts us with reality (we could die at any time and we could die soon), our recognition of our vulnerability creates anxiety and can lead us to wonder if anything we do is meaningful. Thus, Esther appears to be overwhelmed with despair *because* her brother's death confronts her with her own mortality and undermines her sense that her life has meaning. She has abandoned her career and withdrawn into isolation. We do not, at this point, understand her history well enough to know why she was so severely impacted by her brother's death.

Treatment Plan

The Aim

Esther feels alone and without value, but, in fact, her friends continued to care about her and took action to get her help. Their intervention runs counter to her conclusion and points toward one avenue of therapeutic intervention. The sudden loss of her brother left her in mourning (a normal response) but also in despair, as she confronts her own mortality and the meaninglessness (to her) of her life. In order to recover from this double

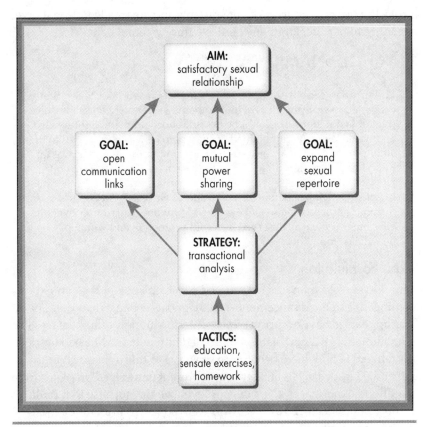

FIGURE 6-7. Transactional category treatment plan (Theresa).

blow, she must not only complete the grieving process but also reestablish her sense of her life's worth and its meaning in the context of her work. That would be the aim of therapy: to reestablish her existential stability.

Goals, Strategies, and Tactics

This aim could be pursued through the person-centered therapy developed by Carl Rogers, an early effort to develop an existential therapy.[4] The goal would be to reexamine her ideas of self and her value system to reestablish her sense of worth and purpose, using Rogers's techniques, such as "being with" the patient and unconditional positive regard. For example, the therapy might focus on the way her teaching activities im-

---

[4]Rogers C: *On Becoming a Person: A Therapist's View of Psychotherapy.* London, Constable, 1961.

prove the careers and lives of her students and create a legacy that gives meaning to her life. Figure 6–8 reflects this system.

PSYCHODYNAMIC CATEGORY

Phillip, a 35-year-old graduate of Harvard Business School, was recently promoted to vice-president of his company. As he entered his new office (bigger and better furnished), he became short of breath, light-headed, and weak. When he complained of chest pain he was transported to the emergency room, but a workup found no cardiac disease, and he was told he had had an anxiety attack. He is the first in his family to go to college. His father, who died last year, worked construction. He had been thinking of his father just before his panic attack. He feels guilty at his "good fortune" of succeeding so far beyond what anyone in his family ever did. He cannot believe he deserved his rapid promotion and wonders when he will be "found out."

Case Formulation

This 35-year-old man had an isolated panic episode in the context of a significant career advancement. The diagnosis is panic disorder. The attack appears to have occurred *because* entering his new office, the tangible embodiment of his new status, confronted him with how he had outdone his father. He may have been more sensitive to this dynamic *because* his father died last year. His anxiety may represent unresolved problems from childhood experiences. On a deeper level, we can surmise that Phillip's anxiety attack occurred *because of* unresolved issues from his oedipal period; for example, his fear of displacing a powerful rival, his father.

Treatment Plan

The Aim

The best outcome might be one that allowed Phillip to put his childhood problems behind him and to function as the adult he now is. This result can be stated as: acceptance of his adult success.

Goals, Strategies, and Tactics

One obvious goal is that he should confront his residual childhood conflict and deal with whatever issues it raises for him in the present. I must consider not only this early conflict, however, but also his relationship with his father, including the impact of his recent death. A second goal, therefore, is the need to reexamine his relationship with his father. Finally, I need to see if his "guilty conscience" is related to other issues in his life; for example, whether his competition for the vice-president position involved behavior he might believe was unethical and therefore a more re-

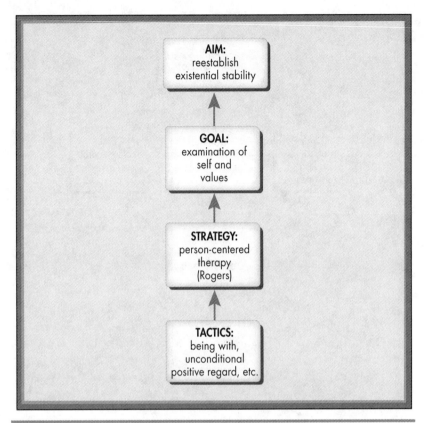

FIGURE 6–8. Existential category treatment plan (Esther).

cent source of guilt. This question of a guilty conscience would form a third goal. I can use a psychodynamic approach to deal with these questions, as reflected in Figure 6–9.

From Treatment Plan to Treatment Contract

It seems self-evident to point out that for a treatment plan to succeed the patient must

1. Know what it is.
2. Agree with it.
3. Be capable of participation in it.

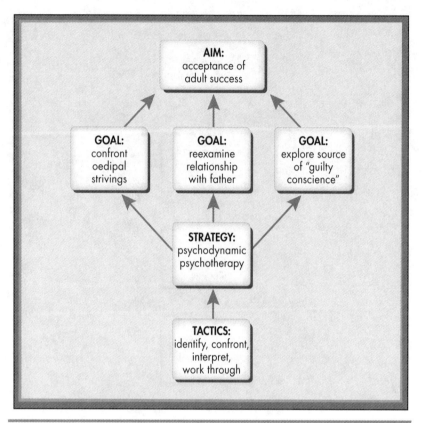

FIGURE 6–9. **Psychodynamic category treatment plan (Phillip).**

So you might reasonably expect that sometime near the end of the evaluation the following steps would occur:

- You, as the architect of the proposed plan, would explain it to the patient.
- The patient would consider the proposal and accept it, ask that it be modified, or reject it.
- If the plan was not acceptable in its original form, the two of you would discuss it further. The discussion would, in fact, be a negotiation and the initial piece of therapeutic work you would undertake.
- You would defend the plan or perhaps change it in response to the patient's objections.
- Both of you would then arrive at a treatment contract that would serve as the basis of the therapy to come.

As sensible as this process may sound, it is remarkable how often it does not take place. It is as if you and the patient collude in an unstated pact that the patient will not inquire and you will not reveal what the treatment will be. Instead, therapy starts off with you in pursuit of your intended goals and the patient responding as best as possible. Sometimes this method works out all right. By happy circumstance the patient's needs and your intentions coincide. After all, even a stopped clock is right…for two seconds every day.

More often, however, the failure to reach agreement results in a gradual divergence of what you want to do and what the patient needs and wants done. In that case, treatment progress slows and finally stops. The therapy devolves into indiscriminate discussions and useless interventions. The two of you can limp along like this for a good while. You may tell yourself you are doing "supportive therapy," and the patient may be satisfied with "venting" or using you as a "sounding board." Unfortunately, whatever problems the patient came to treatment to solve do not get better and the ultimate result is a treatment failure.

SOURCES OF FAILURE

The origin of this failure may be a covert disagreement about the therapy outcome, the aim. You may have a clear idea of what the best outcome of treatment should be. At least, you should hope you do. If that idea is one the patient does not understand or accept, the two of you will work at cross-purposes. Therapy results depend on an active collaboration that can only occur if you both work toward the same result. If not, it usually dooms the treatment.

The basis for the failure can also be at the level of the goals you have set. The source of the disparity between your ideas of what the patient should accomplish and the patient's own ideas about it may originate in the failure to answer the third key question from the initial evaluation: what does the patient want?

- If that question is not answered in the assessment process, your plan will not take it into account.
- If you know what the patient wants but your plan ignores this request, the patient will be unhappy with the therapy direction, even if other worthwhile issues are being addressed.
- If you include what the patient wants in the plan but ignore it in the therapy, the patient will again feel frustrated by the treatment process.

A third source of treatment failure arises from a disagreement about methodology, the treatment strategy. What we ask the patient to do varies a great deal from one methodology to another. Consider the difference between telling patients to talk about whatever is on their mind and instructing them to do a particular behavioral exercise. Patients usually arrive with a set of expectations, derived from a previous experience in therapy or something they have read, heard, or seen, and they will not easily tolerate an unexpected therapy process. In most therapies we ask patients to endure a certain amount of emotional discomfort in the service of healing. It is harder for someone to go through such an ordeal without understanding why it is necessary or how it is supposed to help them.

NEGOTIATION

The effort invested to seek an agreement with the patient is a worthwhile use of therapy time. How long a discussion might be required will vary. With some patients agreement is easily reached, usually by the end of the initial interview. With others it can be a drawn-out process. A patient with strong obsessional traits, for example, may require a nitpicking discussion of details that simulates a legalistic debate, so that it becomes necessary to deal with the patient's style before you can settle on the substance of the plan.

However long it takes, the process is one of proposal and counterproposal. After you explain what you think is going on—in other words, tell the patient your formulation—and answer any questions about it, the obvious next step is to discuss what to do about it. How detailed to make your description of the plan is a matter of judgment, but certainly enough must be said so that the patient understands what the therapeutic task will be and how together you will undertake it. This explanation usually includes a brief idea of the aim, a discussion of the goals, and probably a preliminary description of the methodology. Further education about the therapeutic process will emerge as the treatment proceeds, either by example or by direct instruction, depending on the modality used.

In addition to the specifics of the proposed therapy, the discussion will also include, even if only by implication, the introduction of the healing aspects of psychotherapy that Jerome Frank identified as myth and ritual. The terms are somewhat unfortunate in that they imply "fairy tale" and "unthinking formula."

- Even though we call process "myth," that does not make it untrue
- Even though we label procedure "ritual," that does not mean it is ineffective.

On the contrary, were it not for the powerful influence of myth and ritual in the healing process, psychotherapy would be a lot less successful.

Time Factors in the Treatment Plan

In addition to decisions about what the therapy should accomplish, its main objectives, and the methodology selected, the final plan must also include considerations about time:

- Will the treatment be time-limited or open-ended?
- Will the sessions be closely scheduled or infrequent?

How long the treatment will last may depend on external factors, such as the patient's financial resources or the limitations imposed by a health insurance policy. If these restrictions are present, the treatment plan may need to be modified. Perhaps

- The outcome sought should be more modest.
- The goals should be reduced in number.
- The strategy should be one of the brief therapy methods.

If the limitation is imposed by the patient's life circumstance, the plan may also need to be revised. For example, a schoolteacher who travels abroad each summer will need a more modest plan than if treatment can proceed without interruption. The limitation might also be imposed by the therapist. For example, in a brief therapy protocol, you could set a limit of three or four sessions.

Assuming that sufficient money and time are available, the plan should also include a determination about the frequency, and therefore the intensity, of the sessions. The standard interval, at least in today's third-party environment, is one session per week. On that schedule, the therapy will nevertheless have a constant daily hold on the patient's inner mental life.

- Patients often think about their next meeting with you during the entire interval between sessions.
- They may imagine dialogue and try to anticipate your response to topics they decide to bring up.
- They may brood about whatever was said in the previous session.
- These interval ruminations are often accompanied by strong emotional reactions that may or may not emerge when the next session takes place.

- During these treatment periods, as a result of the emotional intensity of the work and the patient's preoccupation with it (and as surprising as you may find it), you may be the most important person in the patient's life.
- If the sessions are scheduled at greater or less than weekly intervals, some of this intensity will change. Oddly, more frequent sessions do not increase the intensity in proportion. In other words, a twice-weekly schedule does not double it, although it may increase it a bit.
- More frequent sessions will, however, increase the transference feelings that develop in the patient. As the schedule leaves less and less time for events in the patient's real life to intrude, the content of the session becomes more narcissistic and introspective. Thus, a psychoanalysis schedule of four or five sessions a week tends to maximize the intensity of the transference.
- As sessions *decrease* in frequency, however, the effect on the intensity is more marked.

  ➢ When the schedule moves to every other week, for example, with more time for intercurrent events to distract and impinge, the intensity will drop off and the patient will more likely be sidetracked from the work by the intrusion of these extra-therapeutic happenings.
  ➢ At once a month, the need to maintain continuity from one session to the next becomes more difficult.
  ➢ If the patient is seen less often still, it may no longer be possible to prosecute the planned treatment, and the importance of the therapy and your impact on the patient's life will fade, along with the possible benefits of the treatment.

- Another variable in the frequency of visits is the therapeutic benefit of whatever was done in the preceding session. Between one session and the next the patient continues to process the material discussed and the results achieved. These effects percolate through the week and both deepen the therapeutic benefit and prepare the way for the next session's work. As the appointments move closer together, the opportunity for this processing to take place decreases. Therapeutic gains will have less carry-over benefits.
- In addition, in some therapies, such as CBT, the patient is assigned homework between appointments and needs sufficient time to complete it properly.

- These effects are also seen when changes in the schedule result from the patient's attendance.
  - ➤ Patients may cancel their appointment, sometimes more than once, with the de facto schedule going from a reasonable weekly visit to an unworkable, spotty pattern.
  - ➤ External reality may alter the schedule, as when a patient must travel frequently for work or suffers an illness. While these disruptions are often presented as out of the patient's control, they still might be implicated in the patient's efforts to avoid the therapy.
- If these interruptions cannot be dealt with in the therapy, as a resistance to treatment, the plan will need to be revised or, in some cases, abandoned.

Therapy Guidelines

Now that you have completed your initial evaluation, formulated the case, devised a treatment plan, and negotiated a workable treatment contract, you can begin the work of the therapy. Your contract may have included a time limitation, but usually it does not. When a patient asks you, "How long will this take?" the best answer you can give is, "The shortest possible time." In order for that answer to be more than a clever evasion, the therapy has to meet two criteria. It must be

1. *Efficient.* You try to make the greatest possible progress in each session in pursuit of the goals you set in your treatment plan.
2. *Effective.* You try to use the techniques best suited to the problem at hand.

In other words, you try to make every session count. However: "the best laid schemes o' mice and men/Gang oft agley," and in the course of psychotherapy various obstacles will arise to frustrate your efforts. Some of these impediments are discussed below and in the following two chapters.

Treatment Plan Problems

Once the therapy begins, you must

- Avoid a structural impasse.
- Monitor therapy progress.

- Revise the plan when new information emerges.
- End the treatment at the most opportune moment.

THE STRUCTURAL IMPASSE

A structural impasse describes a course of treatment in which progress stops and the therapy is unable to advance despite the best efforts of you and the patient. You may continue to meet and go through the motions, but without any further improvement. In the early going, therapy may seem to make reasonable progress, only to slow and falter at a later point. Enthusiasm wanes, hope fades, and the therapy then either

- Limps along without further progress, leading to an interminable stalemate, or
- Ends with a patient drop-out.

This pattern—a good beginning followed by progressive deterioration— signals a structural impasse. The source of these setbacks is usually to be found in the treatment plan (Table 6–2):

- The treatment plan has been incomplete or omitted altogether.
- The therapy lacks a selected outcome, either because no aim was chosen or because it was inadequately conceived.
- Therapy objectives are poorly selected, with irrelevant, unrealistic, or counterproductive goals.
- You and the patient have not agreed on important methodological questions.
- You and the patient have failed to negotiate a treatment contract.

The solution to an impasse requires the correction of the underlying problem.

- If you have skipped the treatment plan or have only a fragment of one, go back to your formulation and design a new one.
- If you do not have an outcome or you have chosen an inappropriate aim, reexamine the plan and define the desired treatment result more accurately.
- If your therapy goals are poorly defined, rethink what you want the therapy to accomplish and set new goals to reflect these changes.
- If you do not have a treatment contract, negotiate an agreement with the patient about the plan objectives and methodology.

Best of all, put the work into the treatment plan before you start the therapy and avoid these problems altogether.

TABLE 6–2. The structural impasse

Source	Remedy
No treatment plan	Construct a top-down plan
No designated outcome	Complete a formulation, select optimal result
Incomplete treatment plan	Add or delete goals, decide on methodologies
Poorly defined therapy goals	Reexamine formulation, select or modify treatment objectives
Failure to negotiate contract	Educate patient, seek agreement on aim, goals, methods
False agreement	Reopen negotiation, seek valid contract

MONITOR PROGRESS

When you developed the treatment plan, you set up the goals and selected the methods that together would achieve the best outcome. Now, as therapy proceeds, you need some way to know that you and your patient are on the right track and are making progress toward those objectives (Table 6–3). You will have a general sense of progress or the lack of it, but in order to correct interim problems you may need more objective measures.

Problems With Goals

Although you set one or more goals for the therapy, between the initial effort and their final realization you may be able to identify some interim achievements that will tell you that you remain on track to reach your objectives. The interim objectives act as benchmarks to indicate the partial completion of each portion of the plan.

As an example, consider the treatment plan for David,[5] who developed a depression after a broken engagement. Two of the goals were: alleviate depressive symptoms and reverse depressive cognition. To monitor these goals, you can consciously "score" each session: Is he eating and sleeping better? Have the suicidal thoughts declined? Disappeared? Have his automatic thoughts recurred? You could even administer a standardized depression inventory at each session. If he continues to make progress on these measures, the same treatment can continue. If not, something different will be needed.

---

[5]See pages 192–193.

Problems With Process

Every methodology has a process, a way of dealing with the patient's problems that sets it apart from other therapies.

- In a directive therapy, for example, your agenda for each session might include a review of how well the patient fared with the assigned homework since the last session.
- In an exploratory therapy, you might remind the patient of the main topic discussed in the last session and ask for an update.

If you notice that the usual procedure is evaporating and that the effort to use the session to pursue a specific goal has become diffuse, just the recognition of the problem may allow you to correct course and get back on track. Sometimes, however, you need a specific marker, a signpost, as a way to measure progress.

In the above examples, if the patient has not done the homework or if your invitation to pick up the discussion from the previous session is declined, your plan is off track. Even if you do not have an agenda but the patient has nothing meaningful to say, you will realize that progress has slowed. To state the obvious: if you do not monitor progress, you will not know when a therapy problem needs your attention. That problem is likely to worsen and at some point it will threaten to impede the therapy and perhaps will have progressed to a degree that is beyond fixing. These relatively minor problems—a missed homework assignment, a session of off-topic material—are important signs, helpful straws in a disruptive wind, that allow you to deal with threats to progress when they are most manageable.

TABLE 6–3.   Monitor progress

Area of concentration	Focus	Markers	Examples
Outcome of therapy	Interim treatment objectives	Benchmarks	Symptom resolution, behavior change
Process of therapy	Methodology	Signposts	Avoidance, transference, behavior change

REVISE THE PLAN

During the assessment period you gathered enough information to put together a formulation that was the basis of your treatment plan. As therapy progresses you are certain to learn additional history and to make observations that might cause you to modify your formulation and to revise the treatment plan (Table 6–4). These revisions, sort of mid-course corrections, will keep your plan consistent with the facts and relevant to the patient's needs. The new formulations represent successive approximations of the truth, and the revisions recognize the new reality.

- Although unusual, the development of a new and unexpected set of problems may necessitate a new plan and require a change of the aim.
- The emergence of new problems, or new aspects of existing problems, may involve a reevaluation of the objective necessary to bring about the desired therapeutic outcome, a change of goals.
- Alterations in the patient's underlying symptoms and reassessment of the patient's capabilities may demand a shift from one methodology to another, a change of strategy.
- Recognition that a technique is less effective than you expected may require a change of tactics.

In making any of these revisions, you must still follow the top-down approach. That means, if you conclude the plan should be revised,

1. You first consider if you should modify the desired outcome or even select a new one.
2. You next question whether you should alter, delete, or add a goal.
3. If not, you can then reexamine your choice of methodology.
4. And, finally, you can consider using a different technique.

As an example, we can look at our second case of treatment planning: the dilemma faced by Dennis over the decision to get married.[6] The plan contemplated that we help him make a successful transition to adulthood through the use of cognitive therapy to resolve his doubts about marriage, overcome his fear of eventually becoming a parent, and gain some emotional distance from his own parents.

---

[6]See pages 194–197.

- If we discover, after several sessions, that Dennis is reluctant to leave his parents' home because his mother has just been diagnosed with breast cancer and his father's business is failing, our therapy aim could change to "accept existential losses."
- If Dennis reveals that his fear of becoming a parent has concealed the fact that he has an out-of-wedlock child by another woman, our goal might change from "overcome fear of parental responsibility" to "clarify his parental status with his fiancée."
- If our cognitive therapy work created opposition and lack of cooperation because of what we discover is Dennis's obsessional personality traits, we could change our methodology to a psychodynamic therapy.
- If cognitive therapy seemed to be working but Dennis failed to carry out homework assignments, we could abandon that technique in favor of, say, imagery-based exposure.

TERMINATION

I noted in Chapter Three how hard it can be for the patient to leave at the end of a session.

- The patient's dependency needs may fuel efforts to extend the session time and prolong contact with you.
- Separation anxiety and feelings of loss make it harder for the patient to break off contact, even if only for a week.

Imagine how much harder it is, then, to terminate a successful therapy, and how much more strongly the patient may resist it.

Ending therapy can often be fraught with difficulty for you as well. The treatment plan should help make this decision, since when the patient has reached the goals set in the plan, and thereby accomplished the desired outcome, logic would dictate that the therapy is over. Instead,

- As the work seems to approach the goals set at the beginning, new and worthwhile tasks may have evolved and demand attention.
- The comfortable relationship achieved by you and the patient may be difficult to give up.
- It is hard to know just exactly when the original problems have been solved, since remnants of the old behavior remain.
- External forces, such as third-party restrictions, may impinge on your clinical judgment of when therapy should end.

TABLE 6–4. Plan revisions

Focus	Reason for change	Process	Result
Final outcome (aim)	New formulation	Reformulate	New desired result
Plan objectives (goals)	New history and observations modify causation	Add new goal or replace existing goal	Modified plan
Methodology (strategy)	Slow progress, increased dysfunction, new treatment problems	Evaluate each goal, determine best modality	Shift in therapeutic methods
Techniques (tactics)	Resistance, transference, lack of response	Shift technical interventions	Altered therapy technique

The first step in solving these difficulties is to have a commitment to termination and to recognize that

- The patient will continue to benefit from the work you have done even after the final session. Changes and forces set in motion by the therapy will persist, and some continuing gains will even occur more readily without the pressures of the therapy sessions.
- It is in the patient's best interest to end therapy and proceed without your further assistance.

From this philosophical stance you can make good decisions about whatever issues threaten to delay termination (Table 6–5):

- If new problems deserve further therapy you can devise a fresh treatment plan, negotiate a new contract, and begin a new period of therapy aimed at this different outcome.
- Self-examination will help you relinquish a comfortable relationship with a seasoned patient and prepare you to take on the rigors of a new case.
- Recognition that the perfect should not be the enemy of the good—that the patient has achieved the maximum benefits of therapy—will allow you to end treatment when some vestiges of the problem remain.
- Sometimes you must consider your therapeutic ethics and reduce your fees or otherwise modify the business side of the relationship when external forces threaten to terminate treatment prematurely.

Clinical Example: Sally and Julia

In Chapter Four,[7] the initial interview our therapist, Sally, had with her new patient, Julia, ended with a decision to begin weekly sessions to "look for an answer to what you should do with your life." This aim was based on a "developmental" formulation; namely, that Julia had completed her years of child-rearing and homemaking and now faced a new phase of adult development, a period of independence and promise about which she seemed confused and apprehensive. In addition, Julia harbored a core belief that "I'm no good," and she had only limited social support: her increasingly indifferent husband, Hank, and her neighbor,

---

[7]See pages 131–142.

TABLE 6–5. Termination checklist

Conditions	Stop if
Have all therapy objectives been met?	Yes
Has patient reached maximum benefits of treatment?	Yes
Have new problems emerged that require additional treatment?	No
Does a comfortable relationship with the patient challenge the decision to stop?	No
Do external factors (time, money) require premature termination?	No
If external factors are present, can they be overcome?	No

Betty. Although Sally was vague in describing her proposed therapy ("We meet once a week and talk about those ideas and see how it goes."), she may have had in mind a directive strategy. If we put these ideas into a planning diagram, it would look like Figure 6–10.

Later in the therapy, Sally's incomplete treatment contract could cause an impasse as the initial enthusiasm waned and Sally's plan and Julia's expectations diverged. If Sally had been more specific and overt in her negotiation, the interview might have ended with a more satisfactory agreement, as the following transcript shows.

Sally	Let me tell you how things look to me so far, and then we can talk about what to do about it. I think you've come to a point in your life where you're finishing one phase, the part where you raised your girls. They're beginning to make their own way now and they'll need you less than they did before.
Julia	Maybe they won't need me at all.
Sally	I doubt that, but wouldn't you feel good about knowing they could build on all the things you've given them over the years?
	Sally challenges the negative overgeneralization both as a test of her hypothesis and as a test of the therapeutic approach she hopes to use.

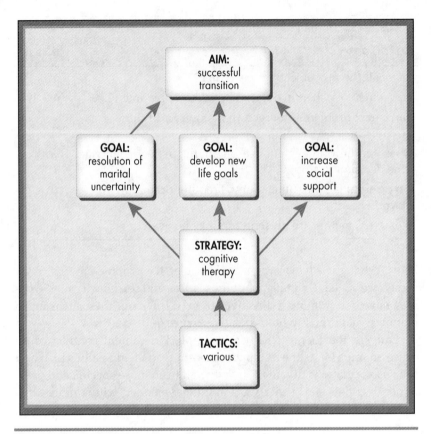

FIGURE 6–10. Planning diagram: Julia.

Julia	I guess so. When you put it that way.
	Julia's response is half-hearted, an early hint of future resistance.
Sally	I think what we should try to do in our therapy work is to look for an answer to what you should do with your life from now on. It seems to me that that's the basic question you're facing. What do you think?
	Sally advances her idea of the aim of the therapy.
Julia	I think you're right, but what about me and Hank?
	Again Julia agrees but may not have entirely accepted Sally's premise.

Sally	That's certainly part of what you need to decide, but I don't think that's the whole story. You also need to look beyond the marriage, whatever you decide to do about it, and consider what your personal goals should be. And also, you seem very isolated. It would help to widen your social circle, to have more people in your life than just Hank and the woman across the street.

> *Sally agrees with Julia's need to make a decision about her marriage, as that seems to be the clearest idea she has about what she wants, and mentions the third goal as well.*

Julia	Okay, that makes sense.
Sally	The approach I'd like to use is called "cognitive therapy." Have you heard anything about that?
Julia	No, I don't think so.
Sally	The basic idea is that how we think about things influences how we feel. For instance, your idea that you mentioned before, that thought that you keep having, "I'm no good," makes you feel depressed and discouraged. You've decided how things will turn out before you've even given them a try. We call those ideas "automatic thoughts," and we need to look into how you came to think that way and whether it's always true or even not true at all.

> *Sally describes a basic tenet of the planned therapy and thus introduces the "myth" of the proposed treatment.*

Julia	And how am I supposed to stop thinking like that?
Sally	We'll take a close look at it and see if we can figure out where it came from and what triggers it the most. I'll suggest some specific ways you can stop it from happening. I might ask you to try certain things between visits and I can give you some material to read, too.

> *Sally describes some of the techniques she might use and thus introduces the "ritual" of the therapy.*

Julia   I thought you were going to ask me questions
             about my childhood. Toilet training and all that.

> *Julia's idea reflects a popular concep-*
> *tion of psychotherapy, perhaps from her*
> *exposure to various media, and gives*
> *Sally a chance to correct her expecta-*
> *tions.*

Sally   That's a different approach, but we might look at
             the experiences that shaped how you think about
             things today. I don't believe toilet training will be
             on the agenda. So, how does all this sound to you?

> *Sally wants to hear if Julia has any ob-*
> *jections or reservations, but otherwise*
> *looks for an overt agreement.*

Julia   It sounds okay. I'd like to give it a try.

At this point Sally and Julia appear to have a therapy agreement. It
will allow them to begin work and also serve as a reference point if problems arise later on.

Key Points

- A complete treatment plan includes
  - ➤ The aim: the desired and optimal outcome
  - ➤ Goals: treatment objectives needed to achieve the desired outcome
  - ➤ Strategies: one or more methodologies selected to fulfill the chosen objectives
  - ➤ Tactics: a selection of relevant techniques for each methodology
- Top-down decisions (first, the aim; then, the goals; lastly, strategy and tactics) are needed to form a workable plan.
- Bottom-up therapy—the use of random strategies and tactics with-out predetermined goals—usually results in diffuse, meandering, and unsuccessful therapy.
- Planning decisions should be based on the case formulation.
- A treatment plan is the basis for negotiation with the patient about what the aim and the goals will be and how the work of therapy will proceed under a treatment contract.

- The plan should be monitored closely to make sure the work proceeds along the lines of the agreement.

- When progress stops—a structural impasse—the reason is usually a problem with the treatment plan. To overcome the impasse, the plan should be revised.

- New information or unexpected developments may require revision of the plan. Aim, goals, strategies, and tactics might need reconsideration and change.

- Therapy should end when the goals are met and the desired outcome is reached.

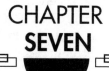

CHAPTER
SEVEN

What Is Communication?

It takes two to speak the truth—one to speak and one to listen.

Henry David Thoreau

It was impossible to get a conversation going. Everybody was talking too much.

Yogi Berra

Introduction

This chapter and the next examine some specific considerations in the conduct of therapy, emphasizing generic techniques and technical considerations, aspects that are not necessarily part of a particular methodology. These general principles and tactics will be useful whatever the goals and strategies selected for a desired outcome and have more to do with common interactions between you and the patient than with the customs and practices of a specific psychotherapy. The focus in this chapter is on the way effective communication can support progress in treatment.

Therapeutic communication always has a purpose:

- To support the therapeutic alliance
- To identify and illuminate areas and topics of significance
- To overcome resistance
- To facilitate behavioral change

You would naturally like your therapy to advance smoothly from session to session until you have accomplished exactly what you and your patient have set out to do. Progress is almost never smooth, however, no matter how skilled and experienced you may be and no matter how motivated the patient is to succeed. The final common pathway of any therapy effort is that patients change their behavior, but that turns out to be one of the most difficult things you could ask of anyone. Behavior seems to (metaphorically) follow Newton's first law of motion: a body at rest tends to stay at rest and a body in motion tends to stay in motion. This inertia will persist "forever" unless an external force acts on it. Your job is to mobilize and direct the therapeutic force that brings about a desired change. Your success in that endeavor depends in large measure on how you minimize or bypass your patients' reluctance, their behavioral inertia, to change in a therapeutic direction.

Communication is the technical skill that implements the treatment plan. If you are to function as a therapeutic instrument, communication will be the change agent, whether it is

- Verbal—the actual words you say to the patient.
- Nonverbal—your tone, expression, posture, and other modifiers.
- Symbolic, as expressed through the setting and your dress and demeanor.

Sometimes more can be conveyed by a lifted eyebrow than by a paragraph of verbiage. Whatever theory or school of psychotherapy you implement, the communicative process conveys that methodology to the patient. In short, to be an effective therapist you must be a communication expert and pay as much attention to this skill as an artist does to the physical characteristics of light and color, an attorney to the legal consequences of each written word, or a surgeon to operative technique. Each of the topics reviewed can, in this brief format, be merely identified and briefly discussed. In-depth exploration of any of them will require further study.

Less Can Be More

As a general rule, the less you say, the more influential each statement, question, or observation becomes. This enhanced significance is perhaps seen most strongly in classical psychoanalysis: when the analyst speaks so rarely—say, perhaps, on an average of once a month—the weight of each pronouncement is greatly magnified. Even in a less drastic system, however, your judicious use of speech can magnify its effect. The patient is more likely to remember, and to be influenced by, a single trenchant observation than by a long exegesis or a wordy explanation. A single question or comment can succeed where a lecture would fail.

That being said, sometimes you must be both active and interrogative, so that you could contribute as much to the dialogue as the patient. This type of enquiry occurs in the service of gathering evidence and is especially important when you attempt to develop the full story. In pursuit of more data you trade the influence that derives from saying little for the usefulness of a more complete understanding. As we'll see in the next section, those efforts are best pursued through a series of questions and only occasionally include direct statements from you.

For most of an average session, your principal occupation is active listening. This effort requires

- *Sustained attention.* Your sole focus is the patient and the here-and-now, not your last session or your next or what you might have for lunch.[1]
- *Eye contact.* To be fully engaged, you must maintain subjective contact with the patient.
- *Awareness of nonverbal as well as verbal communication.*
- *The use of the "observing ego."* You not only listen and observe but simultaneously evaluate and question and then coordinate what the patient says with everything you know.

Then, having collected sufficient data, you can ask a pertinent question or make a helpful observation that will advance the therapeutic agenda. As noted, the more you listen and the less you intervene, the more significant your contribution will be. The decision about when and how to intervene requires the exercise of clinical judgment and will differ in each therapeutic situation.

- In a directive therapy, where assignment of tasks and other instructions are needed, in addition to seeking information on which to base those interventions, you must be more verbally active. This activity must be *in addition* to your active listening and not instead of it.
- In exploratory therapies, less verbal activity is required because you need to hear as much as possible about a topic before coming to a useful conclusion. Nevertheless, your relative passivity should not conceal your interest and concern, attributes you would convey by your nonverbal behavior, such as facial expression and posture.

---

[1]If you do find yourself mentally distracted, consider whether the patient intends (deliberately or unconsciously) to subvert your concentration in the service of avoiding some difficult topic. See section on provoked emotion in Chapter Eight (pages 274–277).

- In experiential therapies, where you may be more likely to draw on personal experience, verbal activity will fall somewhere in the middle of the other two. Again, however, the less you say, the more impact your verbal contributions will have.

Unintended Influence

Not only because of what you intend to convey, but because your communications are necessarily somewhat limited, the effect of *whatever* you do will be greatly multiplied. The profound influence you exert over the direction of patients' thoughts and the significance of your verbal and nonverbal responses are often underappreciated. A direct inquiry or request for further information to which the patient responds with additional or new information is the most obvious overt indication of your interest, but even very subtle hints will have the power to redirect the patient in the direction he or she thinks you want to go. Patients are often exquisitely tuned to your behavior and will alter their communication based on what they think you do or do not want to hear.

- The patient will respond to a slight change of posture, such as leaning forward, or to a minor fluctuation in facial expression, or even to a shift in eye contact, with increased attention to, or possibly avoidance of, whatever topic was under discussion.
- If the patient believes your expression or other nonverbal behavior indicates your disinterest or dislike of the matter at hand, the patient will change the subject and avoid that topic.
- Patients are sensitive to even the smallest indication of your interest or disinterest. The analyst sitting behind the patient out of sight and *doodling* on a pad will create the impression that he is interested in hearing more, with the sound of the pen on paper signaling (wrongly) to the patient that if it is being written down it must be important.
- Even random and completely arbitrary therapist behavior can control the patient's verbal responses. If, for example, an experimenter arbitrarily clears her throat, perhaps on a predetermined schedule of every seven minutes, a transcript would show that whatever the patient happened to be saying at those seven-minute inflection points would become the new and enhanced focus of the patent's discourse, at least for the next seven minutes.

Patients will react to these tiny hints even if they are inadvertent or if you are oblivious to them. This enormous impact means that you should make every effort to be aware of your unintended effect on what your patient talks about. If you notice a seemingly abrupt alteration of topic or an unusual increase to a patient's attention to a subject, think first about how you might have stimulated it. If you believe the change is unwarranted or not useful, you can ask the patient about it and perhaps correct the misinterpretation.

In summary, you want to

- Limit your communication to make it more effective.
- Be aware of how you influence what the patient talks about.
- Minimize the unintentional influence of your behavior.
- Use your influence in a conscious effort to focus the treatment on topics of importance.

An important function of your observing ego is to monitor your own responses, attitudes, and feelings so that you not only pay attention to what the patient says and does but also are fully cognizant of your own contributions. When you are self-aware in your communication, you are at your most effective.

Metacommunication

Communication is a transfer of information between one person (the sender) and another (the recipient). In therapy, as in most communications, this transfer often contains more than one meaning and sometimes an entire hierarchy of meanings. What the patient says to you will have a denotation—the direct meaning of the words—and a connotation—additional information to tell you how those words should be received and interpreted. The extra meanings may be conveyed by the statement itself; for example, by the arrangement of words or by the diction, the choice of which words are used. More often, however, the connotation resides in the nonverbal portion of the communication: the tone of voice, facial expression, word stresses, gestures, and so on. In addition, the words are spoken by the sender to the recipient for a particular reason. The overt purpose is to convey some specific information, but the covert purpose may be a lot more complicated (Table 7–1).

TABLE 7–1. Types of communication

Type of statement	Level of meaning	Use
Denotation	Concrete definitions	Conveys factual information
Connotation	Modified by context	Explains motivation
Metacommunication	Modified by intent	Pursues purpose of statement

LEVELS OF COMMUNICATION

Another way to think about this indirect communication is as a series of levels.

- The literal meaning of the words is the lowest level. No other information is available to understand the statement than the dictionary definition of each of the words used and the context in which the statement is made. For example, "I'm thirsty" means one thing if made in the desert and another if made at a picnic. Its meaning changes with the sentence added: "Do you have any Coke?" and the sentence, "I want to learn everything I can."
- The second level adds the connotation supplied by nonverbal data that is transmitted at the same time. "I'm thirsty" said weakly by a man sweating and breathing hard is a different message from "I'm thirsty" said with a wink and a laugh by a woman in a bar.
- The third level is the reason the statement was made: why were these words said with that connotation at this time? The literal meaning of the words and the additional nonverbal modifiers may be irrelevant. For example, two men at a beer party discussing basketball may actually be engaged in a covert struggle over social dominance (Who is more knowledgeable? Whose team is better? Who has season tickets? and so on). What is important is the motivation and purpose for which the words are uttered at that moment. In the example above of "I'm thirsty," why does the speaker want the hearer to know he or she is experiencing thirst? What does the speaker try to provoke, what response is expected, and why was the information offered at that moment? The term for this third level is *metacommunication*: communication about communication.

   Figure 7–1 illustrates how a metacommunication response shifts the discussion to a new topic.

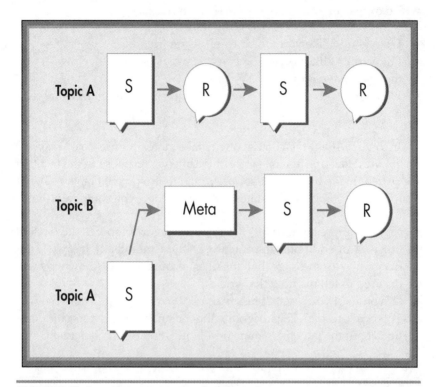

FIGURE 7–1. Metacommunication.
S=sender; R=recipient; Meta=metacommunication.

Connotation

As a simple example, consider how the connotation of a three-word sentence, **I like you**, changes with each of the words stressed:

- **I** like you. (At least I do, even if others don't.)
- I **like** you. (I don't hate you, but I don't love you either.)
- I like **you**. (But not some others I could mention.)

The meaning changes again with nonverbal qualifiers: "I like you" can be said with sarcasm or with sincerity; it can be said tearfully or with a smile, with a wink, with a frown, with a shrug, with raised eyebrows, and so on. The number of permutations for this simple statement is large and varied. Each alteration revises the connotation of the words, and each would require a different response. If you replied, "I like you too," the significance of your response would be different depending on which of the above statements you responded to:

- **I** like you. "I like you too" means we are friends.
- I **like** you. "I like you too" means "I have no stronger feeling for you than you have for me."
- I like **you**. "I like you too" means "we have a more than casual relationship."

In therapy, however, you can often make more progress if you respond on the third level, with a metacommunication: a response to the fact that the patient made the statement rather than to its content (Table 7–2). For example, in response to the statement, "I like you," you could say:

- "Tell me more about that." This neutral answer ignores the content but asks for additional information on the same subject. It says, "I understand your message that you like me, but I want to know why you decided to tell me now that you do."
- "I wonder if you say that because you think it's what I want to hear." This active response again ignores the content but raises a specific question about the patient's timing and motivation for the statement.

TABLE 7–2. Connotation and metacommunication

Example	Connotation response	Metacommunication response
I like **you**. (sarcasm)	Yeah, right!	You don't sound like you mean that.
I like **you**. (sincere)	I like you, too.	I guess you want me to believe you.
I like **you**. (tearful)	Don't cry.	You seem upset

USING METACOMMUNICATIONS

A metacommunication is a response to the implication of a communication rather than to its concrete message. You focus on the meaning of the communication rather than the actual words. You avoid the less useful interaction of a conversation, an apology, a discussion of the substance, or any other type of information transfer that would usually characterize a nontherapeutic interaction. You invite the patient to discuss the reasons for the statement rather than its data. This shift of focus often allows the therapy to progress where a conversational reply would not.

Consider the following exchanges:

> PATIENT: You just sit there and you don't say anything! I'm doing all the work here. What do I pay you for?
>
> YOU (*response #1*): That's not true. I've said plenty, but only when I think what I have to say would be useful.
>
> YOU (*response #2*): Let's talk about what you want from me. What kinds of things should I be saying?
>
> YOU (*response #3*): Isn't that the same feeling you have about your wife? That she doesn't pay enough attention to you?
>
> YOU (*response #4*): You sound like you're pretty frustrated with me.

Your first response is a simple statement that attempts to contradict the patient's exaggeration and correct the record, and your second response also focuses on the content of the patient's statement, even though it invites further discussion. Neither of these replies is likely to lead to new, useful material, and they both ignore the patient's feelings about you. In the third response you assume you know what the patient is feeling, and you make an interpretation based on your assumption, but interpreting a feeling that remains unstated means the patient could easily deny it (either to avoid it or perhaps correctly) and the interpretation could go nowhere. The fourth response is a metacommunication: you comment on the nonverbal aspect of the patient's grievance without agreeing or disagreeing with the complaint. In other words, you ignore what the statement says in favor of what it might mean. Your response identifies a possible reason the patient made the statement but does not attempt to answer the patient's complaint. This approach is more apt to yield useful material that may lead to, and support, the interpretation from response #3 or perhaps point to some other conclusion.

You may need a series of metacommunications. Suppose you notice that a patient is constantly argumentative. Whatever you say, the patient challenges and contradicts it. The next time the patient begins to argue,

> YOU (*metacommunication #1*): I've noticed you like to challenge me. You'd rather argue than discuss.
>
> PATIENT: That's not true. I'm not like that at all.
>
> YOU (*metacommunication #2*): See! Now you're arguing about whether or not you argue.

Sometimes a patient will respond to your metacommunication with another metacommunication, but you can always make a statement about the patient's statement. The dialogue then becomes a series of progressive levels of metacommunicative responses, as if the participants were on parallel ladders and each tried to climb one rung higher than the other. If you persist, however, you can usually prevail and create a useful discussion. Consider the example above of the patient annoyed by your silence. Therapist response #4 ("You sound like you're pretty frustrated with me") was the metacommunication:

> PATIENT: You just sit there and you don't say anything! I'm doing all the work here. What do I pay you for?
>
> YOU: You sound like you're pretty frustrated with me. (*Metacommunication rung #1*)
>
> PATIENT: You're ignoring what I said. (*Metacommunication rung #2; not: You bet I'm frustrated*)
>
> YOU: You're not only frustrated with me in general, now you're frustrated by my response. (*Metacommunication rung #3; not: I'm not ignoring you*)
>
> PATIENT: I think you're just trying to dodge my complaint. (*Metacommunication rung #4; not: I am not frustrated*)
>
> YOU: I'd like to hear about your feelings toward me. (*Metacommunication rung #5; not: I'm not dodging anything*)
>
> PATIENT: My feelings? I'm really annoyed you won't answer me. (*The patient now responds to your last statement with a direct answer, not a metacommunication.*)
>
> YOU: I'd like to hear more about why you're angry. (*You can now respond directly in turn, with the focus shifted from the patient's criticism of your silence and the demand for an explanation to the affect behind the complaint.*)

You have usefully redefined the affect as anger rather than mere "annoyance." Because you did not respond on the same level ("I'm not ignoring you," "I'm not dodging your complaint"), you advance the dialogue to focus on the emotions behind the complaint.

In general, then, the persistent use of metacommunicative responses allows you to manage the subject matter of the discussion and to focus the therapy on a more promising topic. Metacommunication is, at bottom, an exercise of the therapist's power. By declining to accept the patient's statement at face value, you maintain control of the dialogue and avoid the patient's effort to direct you. Your exercise of this power is in the service of making the therapy as effective as possible and is therefore in the patient's ultimate best interest.

Some methodologies, of course, would reject this exercise of therapist control in favor of a laissez-faire strategy that would, theoretically, allow significant material to emerge at its own pace and when it was time for the patient to bring it up. Such an approach might be congenial to a psychodynamic or an existential therapist, for example, who would hold that premature intervention by the therapist could impede progress rather than facilitate it. Either therapist might prefer to meet the patient's complaint with silence or a question. The decision on how active to be—whether to make use of the inherent power in the therapist's role—is a matter of clinical judgment and, of course, personal style.

Questions, Not Statements

To pursue the meaning of a topic or an issue, the more productive process is to ask questions rather than to make statements (Table 7–3). Whatever the patient's assertion, you ask a question about it and then question the answer and the answer after that until you arrive at a satisfactory understanding. This method is sometimes called *Socratic*, referring to the philosophical inquiries of the fifth-century Greek philosopher who said, "I cannot teach anybody anything, I can only make them think." The Socratic dialogue assumes the questioner knows the answer, even if only in general terms, and uses this technique to lead the student to it. In therapy, however, you may not know the answer or may think you know it only to discover a different or better one. A Socratic dialogue—question, answer, question, answer—is nevertheless often the most useful way to

- Explore complex ideas.
- Reveal underlying assumptions.
- Uncover the facts.
- Analyze problems.

TABLE 7–3. Statements versus questions

Statement	Question
Takes authoritarian stance	Suggests egalitarian effort
Claims expert status	Recognizes equal partnership
Suggests decisive answer	Maintains open-ended inquiry
Assumes definitive conclusion	Acknowledges tentative estimate
Stimulates disagreement	Seeks agreement
Provokes resistance	Invites cooperation

When you ask a question, the patient is

- Invited to participate on an equal footing in the search for understanding.
- Asked to shoulder part of the responsibility for getting to the truth of the matter.
- Discouraged from debate or argument with you.
- Dissuaded from opposing you as a form of resistance.

As an example, suppose a patient tells you his neighbor's dog has been digging up his garden and he wants to shoot it. You could warn him of the adverse consequences of his idea, but consider the way a series of questions helps clarify and resolve the problem:

You	Do you mean that you'd like to shoot it or that you actually intend to do it?
	You ask whether this is a fantasy or a plan. At the same time, simply asking the question raises the possibility that it is not a good idea.
Patient	I'd like to do it, and I will if that animal comes into my yard again.
You	Is that a good idea?
	By using the form of a question, you raise the "good idea" subject directly but without taking a position yourself that could turn into a debate. This question, and the next two, may suggest what your opinion is but they do not excite the same opposition as would a direct statement. Because they do not challenge the patient directly they encourage his participation in the discussion.
Patient	It solves my garden problem.
You	Would it cause you any other problems?
	You invite the patient to think it through.
Patient	(*laughs*) I'd probably get in trouble. Just firing the gun would get me arrested.
You	Is that worth it to you? Solving one problem and causing another?

Patient   No, I guess it isn't. But I'd still like to do it.

> *The patient is unlikely to take action but gives a face-saving answer. No need to take it further and force him to "promise" not to do it.*

You   What makes you so angry about it?

> *Now that the danger is past, you can invite the patient to examine his apparent overreaction.*

Some patients in this situation might accuse you of trying to talk them out of shooting the dog. Even though you do have an opinion—don't shoot the dog—you would explain that

- You are only asking questions.
- The decision is the patient's. Whatever you might do in his situation is irrelevant.
- He will bear the consequences, not you, so it does not matter what you think.

The accusation that you want to talk him out of it might reveal a transference issue: the patient thinks you are autocratic and controlling, or that you look down on him for his anger, or even that you might turn him in to the police if he went through with it. This development would then require an examination of those feelings and could be even more productive. If you had simply told him not to do it, you could not then cite as evidence that you only raised a question, and he took it to mean something worse. Your actual advice, in the form of a statement, would make this task a lot more difficult.

In addition, a series of questions, each one seeking more detail and further clarification, is effective in the effort to get to the core of an issue. Think of how a young child might question every answer and how much information that generates.

—Why is the sky blue?
 —Because the sun shines through it.
—But why does the sun shine?
 —Because it's made of fire.
—But why does fire make light?
 —Because it sends out energy.
—But what's energy?

And so on.

Under ordinary circumstances, only children can ask "endless" questions without social consequences. In an adult conversation, between friends or in any social setting, continued questioning might seem rude, intrusive, overly aggressive. Within the therapy relationship, however, a different set of expectations prevails. The treatment contract empowers you to confront, to question, to challenge, and to intrude, because the inquiry is in the service of healing and done with the patient's agreement. The process is reinforced, for both you and the patient, when it produces helpful material and results in measureable improvement.

The kind of questions that come up in therapy range from simple requests for additional information to probing inquiries into motivations. A sample would include

- *Requests for clarification.* You ask for more information about a topic or an issue.

  ➢ "What did you mean when you said…?"
  ➢ "Can you say more about that?"
  ➢ "Do you mean to say…?"

- *Confirmation inquiries.* You ask about a possible problem or problem area.

  ➢ "Is it difficult for you to…?"
  ➢ "Has that been a problem for you?"
  ➢ "What's in the way of your doing that?"

- *Consideration queries.* You ask the patient to think more carefully or to look at a possible consequence.

  ➢ "Is that a good idea?"
  ➢ "What do you think might happen if…?"
  ➢ "What would you do if…?"

- *Socratic invitations.* You ask the patient to think through a problem.

  ➢ "What does it mean to you when someone says…?"
  ➢ "What is good (or bad) about…?"
  ➢ "What would you do if…?"

- *Why questions.* On many occasions the question that comes to mind might begin with "why." Unfortunately, "why" questions have a built-in difficulty. Although their ostensible subject is motivation, the use of "why" can easily imply criticism. Power in the asymmetric relationship resides more strongly in the therapist, but you should not abuse that power to reproach, disparage, or condemn the patient. For example:

> "Why did you drink last night?"
> "Why did you get into that argument?"
> "Why did you yell at your wife?"

Some why questions, however, can be useful when they are merely inquiries and are more judgment neutral, but the distinction can be difficult to make.

> "Why did you go to Los Angeles?" ("I'm curious about your choice," not "Didn't you know you'd be breaking parole?")
> "Why did you ask about that?" ("I'd like to know more about your interest," not "Don't be rude.")
> "Why does that make you angry?" ("I'm interested in how you feel," not "You're wrong to feel that way.")

• *Cross-examination questions.* If you think you know the answer to some problem or the background of some therapy issue, you can initiate a series of questions designed to confirm or deny your expectation. An attorney questioning a witness attempts to "lay a foundation" by establishing the basis for a fact he wishes to bring into evidence. The foundational questions may at first seem unrelated to the subject but later prove to support the direct question about it. Each question has a single topic of inquiry (rather than compound questions that require several answers). Thus:

> ATTORNEY: You work for the *New York Times*, don't you?
> WITNESS: Yes.
> ATTORNEY: And from time to time you write articles?
> WITNESS: Yes.
> ATTORNEY: And you wrote an article on January 3rd about a New Year's party?
> WITNESS: Yes.
> ATTORNEY: And in that article you said my client was drunk?
> WITNESS: Yes, I wrote that.
> ATTORNEY: Did you ever meet her personally?
> WITNESS: No.
> ATTORNEY: So, you never actually knew if she was drinking or not?
> WITNESS: No.

And so on.

In therapy, of course, you want a collaborative association rather than the adversarial relationship of the courtroom. Collaboration requires that you adopt the lawyer's technique to help you gather information or to make a point, but you avoid the antagonistic attitude. Only the principles would be the same: lay a foundation, approach the topic in small steps, and ask simple questions on a single topic.

> PATIENT: My husband came home drunk last night and I threw a plate at him.
> YOU: Does he often stay out drinking? (*Foundation*)
> PATIENT: No, just once in a while.
> YOU: So that wasn't his typical behavior? (*Confirmation*)
> PATIENT: No.
> YOU: Did you expect him to do it this time? (*Foundation*)
> PATIENT: I had an idea he might. We had a big fight that morning before he went to work. I want to go to a resort on our vacation, and he wants to stay home and putter around the house.
> YOU: And you think he got drunk because of the fight? (*Foundation*)
> PATIENT: It's his typical reaction.
> YOU: Were you still angry from the morning, while you were waiting for him? (*Foundation*)
> PATIENT: Yes, I was. And I got more and more upset when he didn't show.
> YOU: Maybe you two need a better way of settling an argument. (*Conclusion*)

- *Interpretative questions.* Interpretations take many forms and can vary with the methodology you use. An interpretation may present a cause-and-effect connection or an alternative motivation or an unexpected identification. Since you are never certain that the idea you advance in an interpretation is correct, any suggestion of this type is only tentative and can more usefully be presented in the form of a question.

  ➢ "Did you get angry because she reminded you of your mother?"
  ➢ "Do you think you got so angry because you're strongly attracted to him?"
  ➢ "Did she stir up your old anger from when that teacher used to pick on you?"

Asking useful questions is an art. The line between a question that advances the work and one that stirs up unnecessary resistance can be easily crossed. Some patients are exquisitely sensitive to perceived criticism and others are readily moved to argument by any hint of reproach. A question that seems a neutral inquiry to you may wound the patient's narcissism and result in hurt feelings. While any of these reactions would be grist for the therapeutic mill, they may sidetrack an important therapeutic effort and delay progress. To avoid those consequences, you need to be finely attuned to the patient's emotions. Sensitivity and empathy will alert you when the questions you want to ask elicit a different response than you expected or needed. At that point a metacommunication (for example, "Did my question upset you?") may help to straighten out a misunderstanding.

Veracity and Deceit

Humans are not truthful. Deceit is encoded in our DNA, a survival skill like a chameleon's ability to camouflage itself to hide from its enemies. Humans lie: we dissemble, we fabricate, we misrepresent, we "spin," we prevaricate, we mislead, we "put on a face to meet the faces that you meet." Mothers lie to children and children to their parents, husbands to their wives and wives to husbands, friends lie to friends. Politicians get elected through mendacity, drug manufacturers get rich by quackery, journalists make news out of canards, authors are paid for fiction, retailers profit from falsehoods, lawyers win cases through calumnies. No one tells the truth, the whole truth, and nothing but the truth, even under oath. Everybody lies. It would be a challenge to get through a single day without a lie.

So, you should not be surprised when your patients deceive you.

- They may deliberately tell you something they know to be false.
- They may lie by omission.
- The false narrative may result from unconscious motives.
- The falsehood may be motivated by transference feelings: shame, guilt, fear of retribution.

Absent delusional ideation or irrational belief, patients generally know when they are lying.

Sometimes patients' mistaken view of reality may lead them to say something they believe to be true, although from your point of view or prior knowledge you know it to be false. It is easier to correct a mistake than to challenge a lie, although both may be defended at great length. In either case, if patients behaved without hypocrisy, pretense, duplicity, or misrepresentation, their therapy would be shorter and more successful. Veracity is rare, however, and you are challenged to find what facts you can within the half-truths and prevarications you hear in every session.

Although you must expect to hear a false narrative, you usually should not confront the patient with skepticism or disbelief. If a patient perceives that you doubt or reject what he or she says, the therapeutic alliance will suffer. At the same time, since your task is to uncover the truth behind the patient's behavior, you cannot take everything at face value. To solve this dilemma, you must, as usual, operate on two levels at once.

- Your overt response must be to accept everything the patient says as valid and reliable. Even though this attitude may seem naïve and gullible, you must be attentive, accepting, trusting, and credulous.
- Your covert response, however, must include a skeptical, even suspicious, attitude, one that looks for contradictions, logical inconsistencies, and just plain fibs. The concealed skeptic is one facet of your observing ego, the "inner eye" that continually examines and evaluates what both you and the patient say and do. Through your observing ego you try to identify improbable claims, unlikely narratives, and other evidence of falsehood.

Once having identified these questionable areas, however, it is not usually helpful to challenge the patient directly. Confronted with the uncovering of fabrications, people often lie more and sometimes challenge the questioner to "prove it" or become angry at the supposedly false accusation. In therapy this direct confrontation is not often productive and can even prove harmful. Instead, in the manner discussed in the preceding section, you can approach the issue obliquely or in small steps, first questioning some obvious incongruity, then a more central conflict, until you finally work your way into the heart of the issue. As previously outlined, in this effort you operate somewhat in the manner of a lawyer cross-examining a witness. The lawyer is aware of what testimony she wants to elicit, but she always tries to lay a foundation, so that each question builds on the one before it. She begins at the margins of the evidence and, through a series of questions, moves toward the central facts. In the same way, using a gradual approach and asking questions (rather than making statements), you can achieve successive approximations of the truth. Your ability to find the truth behind the deception often depends on your success in recognizing the inconsistent details and picking away at them until the larger inconsistencies come to light. This effort usually requires an obsessional attention to detail that might be considered a maladaptive trait in ordinary social relations but is a useful tool in the therapeutic context.

For example, suppose your patient, a 14-year-old girl, comes in wearing a neon blue lip color.

PATIENT (*pointing to her lips*): What do you think?
YOU (*to avoid giving an opinion*): Never saw you wear that before. Where did you find it?
PATIENT: My mother gave it to me. It's an expensive brand.
YOU: Your mother wears that color?
PATIENT: No! It was a gift.
YOU: What was the occasion?
PATIENT: No occasion. She saw it in the store and thought I'd like it.
YOU: You said your mother never buys you anything. So this is pretty unusual, isn't it?
PATIENT: You don't believe me?
YOU: Shouldn't I believe you?
PATIENT: She could have bought it for me.
YOU: How did you really get it?
PATIENT: Shoplifting.

Uncovering the lie would then allow the focus to shift to a therapy issue—her relationship with an apparently indifferent mother—that would not have come up if you had merely replied to her initial question, "Very striking," and let the issue go. Even worse would be if you said, "Oh, did you steal that, too?"

Patients' deceptions may be more extensive than the denial or distortion of a single fact. Patients may conceal an entire chunk of personal history or misrepresent an incident or a past experience. They may present themselves in a falsely favorable (or even falsely unfavorable) manner. Their motivation for these distortions may be manipulation or narcissism or feelings of guilt or shame. The effort to get to the truth behind these large-scale deceptions is often the task of a large section of therapeutic work. When you uncover one layer of falsehood, you often find another underneath, so that the therapy is a progression of gradual discovery that eventually leads to the underlying facts.

Rhetoric and Persuasion

Psychotherapy is sometimes described as "talk therapy," but a more accurate definition would be "persuasive talk therapy." Its purpose is always to bring about helpful changes that will correct the patient's dysfunctional behavior, but it has no direct power to modify that behavior. You can only persuade a patient to make the necessary changes. Sometimes a change results from actions you recommend, such as the "homework"

a cognitive therapist might assign, but most often these helpful modifica-
tions follow from the effects of what you say in the session that induces
the patient to act differently. How you say something often determines
its persuasive force. The same observation said in different ways can vary
greatly in how it impacts the patient.

Rhetoric is the science of persuasive speech, a set of skills developed
and taught since ancient times. Aristotle, for example, identified three
persuasive components of rhetorical speech:

1. *Ethos*—the speaker's good character, as evinced by his virtue, intelligence, and goodwill, gives his speech credibility. In therapy, ethos
   arises from the therapeutic alliance between you and your patient.
2. *Logos*—the appeal to logic. The force of this component resides in the
   myth (the theoretical logic of the internal structure of a psychotherapy system) and the ritual (the procedural logic of the methodology
   of the therapy).
3. *Pathos*—the use of storytelling, metaphor, and other figures of speech
   to appeal to the emotions of the listener. This third skill is one that may
   be underappreciated as a therapeutic technique.

From time to time, you will need to convey to your patient an interpretation or observation or conclusion that must be strongly persuasive,
whether it is a major intervention or simply an effort to have what you
say seriously considered. In this effort you can strengthen the impact of
your comments with the rhetorical devices of the "pathos" component.

- Tell a story as a kind of parable or an illustration.
- Use an anecdote to illustrate your point.
- Convey your idea through metaphor.

Sometimes you can use contemporary material to help strengthen
your argument: a scene from a well-known film, the lyrics from popular
music, or other commonly appreciated cultural phenomena. Film and
television, novels and song lyrics, in print or online, both reflect the culture and help shape it. When you illustrate a point by reference to these
fictional media, you not only provide a metaphor but also summon the
persuasive power of cultural expectation. Occasionally a joke might help,
although humor can easily be misinterpreted and should be used with
caution.

As an illustration consider the problem of a pessimistic patient an-
ticipating a bad outcome before the event. You could point out that the

conclusion is premature and that it may turn out well after all. That approach would utilize *logos,* an appeal to logic. You could make a stronger point, however, with something from the *pathos* approach, like the following, "jack story":

> A man is driving late at night on a country road when his car gets a flat tire. He has a spare but discovers he is missing a jack. He recalls that he just passed a farmhouse and decides to walk back to borrow a jack. On the way he thinks, "It's really late. I might have to wake him up." He walks a bit more and thinks, "He's going to be angry about my disturbing him." He walks on, but a few minutes later, he thinks, "I bet that bastard will be so angry he won't want to lend me a jack." He reaches the farmhouse and sees all the lights are out. "He'll refuse to help me," he mutters. "Maybe he'll try to shoot me." He knocks on the door, a light goes on upstairs and the farmer pokes his head out the window, and says, "Yes, can I help you?" "Never mind," the man shouts, as he angrily stalks away, "I don't want your goddamn jack anyway."

The jack story is not inherently significant. It does not contain great characters or a tricky plot. It is not memorable for its wisdom or eternal truths. It is simply a rhetorical device to illustrate an idea: don't let your emotions distort your judgment. Like Aesop's fable of the fox who cannot jump high enough to reach a bunch of grapes and concludes, "Those grapes were sour anyway," it provides a persuasive image for an intangible concept. Aesop's fable persists in the culture, now separated from its origin, as the well-known excuse of "sour grapes." If you used this flat-tire anecdote in a therapy session you might hope that the patient would avoid making emotional prejudgments in the future by thinking, "Oh, that's another jack story."

Rhetorical speech requires us to think harder and more creatively about the best way to communicate our ideas, but the effort is often repaid with a more effective outcome.

Modeling

As a specific technique, modeling is used in certain kinds of cognitive therapy as a method of teaching or reshaping dysfunctional behaviors into more effective ones. In a larger context, however, modeling is a universal human learning process, as reflected in the adage "Imitation is the sincerest form of flattery."

- Children model themselves after parents, teachers, rock stars, and other admired persons, through the process of identification and imitation.

- Adolescents and adults model through a series of *partial identifications*, a process that selects a small piece of behavior—a gesture, a mannerism, a speech pattern, hairstyle, habits, clothing—and incorporates it into an existing identity, often accompanied by some admired basic attribute of the person imitated. Partial identifications can focus on almost anything about another person, provided that the trait or behavior is esteemed and valued, and most of the time the person imitating the other is unaware of it. A partial identification often reflects admiration and respect for the entire person imitated, even though only a portion of that individual's persona is copied. Through partial identifications people adopt the successful habits and strategies of others and thereby become more successful themselves. Sometimes, however, identification leads to the assumption of undesirable behaviors. When a child who is bullied becomes a bully in turn, for example, it reflects a defense known as "identification with the aggressor."[2]

Through partial identification with someone admired,

- A shy person might become more outgoing.
- An unambitious person might strive to succeed.
- An impulsive person might become more thoughtful.
- An independent voter might join a political party.
- An undecided teenager might choose a particular career.

These identifications can also operate in unhappy ways: the teenager might take up smoking or use other drugs or join a gang.

In a psychotherapy environment, modeling is a remedial force at work behind every specific methodology. As a model for the patient, you embody several helpful characteristics:

- You demonstrate a mature mindset—the exploration of alternatives, deferring judgment until all the facts are known, a search for underlying motivation—that the patient can adopt and use independently of the therapy.

---

[2]*Identification with the aggressor* is an unconscious (ego) defense, described by Anna Freud in 1936, that allows a victim to avoid shame and anxiety by "becoming" the person responsible for the (real or perceived) threat, abuse, or assault.

- You maintain an emotional detachment from the upsetting experiences and recollections of the patient. This distance is, of course, generated partially by your observer status, but it also reflects a levelheaded and self-possessed attitude that appeals to a patient roiled by the emotions generated in the therapy. This model is captured in the idea "If it doesn't bother her, why should it bother me?"
- You approach problems from a rational and logical point of view, based on an underlying premise that these issues can be understood and solved by a careful and reasonable approach. This competent stance counterbalances a patient's tendency to feel overwhelmed and helpless in the face of emotional disorder. "If he feels confident we can solve this, I can be too."
- You are nonjudgmental about whatever events and feelings generate shame and guilt in the patient. This accepting attitude encourages the patient to be less harsh in self-judgments. "If she doesn't look down on me, maybe I'm not so bad."
- You convey a positive regard for the patient that, in turn, encourages the patient to adopt a more positive self-assessment. "If he thinks well of me, I must be all right." In patients with a critical, withholding, or rejecting figure in their past, this influence is sometimes called the "corrective emotional experience"[3] that is a general benefit of the therapeutic alliance.

None of these effects is, of course, guaranteed to work to overcome the patient's helplessness, self-criticism, or poor self-image, but your role as a model presents an alternative to the patient's negative judgments.[4] Moreover, they operate continuously in the background without your having to make any overt attempt to convey the ideas they represent.

At times, however, you may be able to make a more deliberate impact on the patient by selectively modeling behaviors that are focused on the personality traits that form a background to the patient's immediate problems (Table 7–4). These behavioral presentations would be separate and apart from whatever therapeutic work was going on under the treat-

---

[3]*Corrective emotional experience* is a concept developed by Carl Rogers, Franz Alexander, and others that describes an important therapeutic mechanism: The reexperience of a past psychic trauma under the safe, nonjudgmental conditions of a benign psychotherapy environment promotes and facilitates healing.

[4]You can model a role, but you are not a "role model" unless your patient is another therapist.

ment contract.[5] You would make a personality assessment, as part of your general evaluation, and be on the lookout for evidence of these traits in the session.

TABLE 7–4. Examples of modeling

Trait	Modeling
Borderline	Affective stability and good impulse control
Dependent	An independent mind set and self-reliance
Obsessional	Flexibility and acceptance of imperfection
Avoidant	Social skills and confidence
Narcissistic	Concern and respect for others

Naming, Renaming, and Reframing

Architecture might be described as the science of defining space. The architect circumscribes an open, unbounded area with construction—walls, floors, roofs of specified sizes and shapes—that confines and constrains empty, unlimited space into a finite structure with a determined use and a specified purpose. In psychotherapy, regardless of the specific methodology, you also define boundaries that allow you to better deal with the behaviors and emotions you want to modify. The act of labeling something that has previously been unnamed gives it a shape, form, and function that allows you to conceptualize it, to understand it, and, if necessary, to alter it. For example: a patient who comes to the doctor with a cough might be worried: "Is this an infection, TB, pneumonia? Is it cancer? Is it fatal?" Once the doctor diagnoses the illness and names it, the patient's worries are relieved. If the news is good ("It's only a cold") or if it is bad ("It's lung cancer"), the previous anxiety created by an unnamed threat dissipates, although other concerns might ensue ("Do I have to miss work?" "Can the cancer be removed?").

NAMING

In psychotherapy, naming can be specific or general, concrete or abstract. If you label a patient's problem with other people as "social anxiety," or you

---

[5]You can sometimes model alternative behaviors for specific disorders. Jay Haley would rub his hand across the sole of his shoe and then over his face and hair when his patient suffered from a fear of dirt and germs.

label a lack of energy and motivation as "depression," you have taken the initial step in the treatment process, not only because you can then construct a plan to deal with it, but, more important, because you have allowed the patient to separate from it. It is no longer the vague idea, "I have problems with other people," but rather "I have social anxiety"; no longer "I have no energy or interest in doing anything," but rather "I'm depressed." The name allows the patient to gain distance from the problem, to view it as something specific that can be dealt with, to avoid the dysphoric state that results from not knowing what is wrong.

You can achieve the same benefit if you name symptoms or conflicts or cognitive errors.

- A frightening experience of dry mouth, pounding heart, and tremors, when named a "panic attack" (and not a heart attack), becomes a manageable problem for which there are short-term fixes (rebreathing from a paper bag) and long-term solutions (exposure and response prevention).
- A series of unsuccessful dating experiences, when named a "fear of commitment" (and not failure due to physical or personal defects), becomes a focus of inquiry and exploration that can lead to a long-term relationship.
- A history of unsuccessful employment, when named the result of "automatic thoughts" (and not laziness or stupidity), becomes the basis for cognitive strategies to deal with "Whatever I try to do I always fail."

The benefits of naming create a strong argument for sharing your formulation with the patient. As discussed in Chapter Six,[6] the formulation is an integral part of treatment planning and should be a part of negotiating the treatment contract. When you tell the patient your formulation, in effect naming the patient's problem, you improve the prospects for a good outcome to the therapy:

- You strengthen the therapeutic alliance by your demonstrated expertise in putting the formulation together.
- You establish that the patient's problems make sense and fit into a coherent explanation of why and how they developed (the myth), thus adding to the patient's confidence in the therapeutic process.

---

[6]See pages 191–192.

- You enlist the patient's collaboration in the work of therapy because you imply that if the problems can be understood, they can be helped (the ritual).

RENAMING

When the patient has already named something, and that name contributes to the patient's problems, you can often help by supplying a new, different name. If you change the name—if you rename the problem—you can begin to alter both the patient's perception of it and its impact. The renaming process often involves the same shift of emphasis as the definition of a glass as half full rather than half empty. For example, the patient says, "I'm too timid. I don't like to make a decision until I'm sure it's the right one, and I miss out on opportunities." If you rename the patient's "timid" as "cautious" or "prudent," you suggest that the trait the patient considers a fault is actually a strength.

When and how to rename a patient's behavior is, of course, a matter of clinical judgment. If the reversal will be useful in the overall therapy, you can then rename the problem. At the least, it helps the patient improve self-esteem and perhaps correct a cognitive distortion, both of which could be useful to the therapy effort. At times, however, the problem should remain a focus of the treatment plan, in which case you can name it, but you should not rename it.

Renaming is also useful if you need to define something the patient does not consider a problem as, indeed, something that needs attention, modification, or therapeutic correction. These ego-syntonic behaviors, when relabeled, are given separation and distance that allows them to become the focus of therapy. Patients might consider themselves, for example,

- Introspective and thoughtful rather than self-absorbed and egotistic.
- Careful and observant rather than nitpicky and perfectionistic.
- Loving and caring rather than overly dependent and clinging.

As the above examples indicate, these behaviors often reflect troublesome personality traits rather than symptoms of a specific disorder. Renaming them will often be perceived by the patient as a narcissistic blow. Careful judgment is required before taking this step.

REFRAMING

The concept of renaming can be expanded to include the larger problems with which patients present. The interpretation is broader and can now be designated as reframing. The concept differs from the "cognitive restructuring" associated with cognitive therapy, which refers to an effort to reverse negative or self-defeating *thoughts*. Instead of changing the label on a single behavior, reframing is the effort to modify the conceptual or emotional aspects of an entire circumstance or pattern of behaviors in order to give it a more useful meaning. The process cuts across methodological lines and offers a general strategy useful in different types of therapy. It may involve

- A single, immediate intervention. For example, an athlete who loses a race might benefit if the result is reframed as a learning experience.
- An extended period of therapeutic work. For example, a patient who escapes a terrorist bombing but suffers from survivor guilt may be helped to recover if the experience is reframed as a social good because of the effect the survivor's death would have had on family, friends, coworkers, and others.

Here is one clinical example. A patient of mine whose marriage was shaky said she felt contempt for her husband because he wasted his musical talents on a local amateur group when she knew he was capable of more professional, high-level achievement. I pointed out that amateur protégés were his only option, that he would welcome a professional chance, but, as she knew, nothing was available to him. Give Picasso a bucket of mud and a bundle of sticks, I told her, and he would create art. In the same way, her husband was doing the best he could with the opportunities available to him. She appeared disconcerted by how I had reframed her assessment and said no more about it, but, much later, she said that my comments had saved her marriage. (Also note how my use of persuasive rhetoric, my reference to Picasso, strengthened my case.)

The task of reframing is the effort to challenge and modify a set of beliefs or self-characterizations that create dysfunction and emotional damage and to provide an alternative, more helpful viewpoint. In this regard you are not merely an apologist or a Pollyanna, but rather a facilitator of the healing process.

Dream Interpretation: Symbolic Communication

In the context of therapy, a dream can usefully be considered as one of the patient's efforts at communication. Unlike waking communications, dreams convey meaning through symbols rather than words. Patients are less likely to tell you their dreams today than they were when "Freud" was synonymous with psychotherapy and everybody knew analysts were always interested in dreams. Nevertheless, some patients will still report a dream, or more often a recurring dream, and expect you to explain it.

Freudian analysis concentrated on dream elements rather than the dream as a whole. The story the patient told about the dream was considered the "manifest content," an attempt to make a coherent narrative out of what was actually a loose collection of symbols and images. This underlying collection was called the "latent content," and the patient was asked to take each of these elements and free associate to it in order to uncover whatever ideas and conflicts it reflected. The theory was that dreams were wish fulfillments that could be reconstructed through this process.

In weekly psychotherapy this method of understanding a dream may not be practical. An alternative method of dream analysis, however, is available (Table 7–5). It accepts the manifest content, the dream narrative as the patient recalls it, as a valid expression of an important issue in the patient's life. The manifest content can often be linked to some contemporary event or problem (what Freud called the "day residue"), and this link can be a starting point to understand the dream. In this approach, you consider the recounted dream as a report from the patient, even if it sounds bizarre and illogical, as dreams usually do. Understanding the dream in this manner is informed by 1) its affect and 2) its theme.

TABLE 7–5.   Dream interpretation

Psychoanalytic	Generic
The royal road to the unconscious	An alternate style of communication
Manifest content has no meaning	Dream tells a useful story
Latent content crucial	Latent content ignored
Dream affect secondary	Dream affect informative
No central theme	Central theme conveys meaning

1. No matter how disguised and symbolically modified the underlying concerns are, the emotion connected to those worries is transmitted without distortion. If the dominant affect is anxiety or anger or sexual excitement, then the dream is about an anxiety-provoking or anger arousing or sexually stimulating subject.
2. The disparate elements in the dream narrative will usually fit within a single category that can be considered the central theme of the dream. To identify the theme, you must, once again, exercise your inductive reasoning as you try to generalize from a collection of particulars. Inductive logic, as we discussed in the chapter on formulation, is a difficult process, but a helpful starting point is the day residue, the events closely preceding the dream night. Also helpful is to link the dream to the patient's main problems, those the therapy is dealing with at the time, on the grounds that those issues will more readily find their way into sleep-generated ideation.

As an example we can return to the patient we met in the second chapter: Matthew, age 24, a graduate student who completed his M.B.A. degree and relocated to start a new job, interrupting his psychoanalysis. He knows no one outside his new office and feels isolated and lonely. He also reports moderate social anxiety, reflected in his worry, "What will people think of me if I let them get to know me?" In his recurring dream, he is in a house, his own home even though he does not recognize it, and strangers are entering the home through flimsy doors and along unguarded hallways. He becomes more and more frantic, trying to close off these points of entry and to keep the trespassers out, but he cannot, and they will not leave.

To understand the dream, you first note that the dominant affect is anxiety, verging on panic. The patient's inability to keep his home safe from intruders suggests the theme is "vulnerability." Based on these two observations, and in conjunction with the available fragment of history about the effect his move has had on his social status, you can surmise that his dream's message is "I can't protect myself against exposure to people in my new environment." At the same time the dream presents him with lots of new people trying to visit him, perhaps reflecting his wish to make new friends and expand his social life. These conclusions might lead to a useful discussion about Matthew's fears and, depending on what type of therapy you thought might be most helpful, a goal to increase his social activity by reducing his irrational fear of rejection.

When you use a dream in this limited way, and view it as a parable or a fable, you can often short-circuit the lengthy path of exploration and get to the heart of the patient's problem more quickly. In the condensed symbolism of the dream, conflicts, fears, and wishes are more readily accessible, and the patient is likely to be more accepting of your ideas because, after all, you are talking about something the patient produced and asked you to interpret. As every instance from Pharaoh's dream in the Old Testament to nightmares in modern novels demonstrates, when you are the author of the dream, you are predisposed to believe in its meaning.

Final Thoughts

Communication is the fundamental instrument of every psychotherapist. In metaphorical terms, it is the river over which the methodological boats must travel. Whether the boat is labeled psychodynamic or cognitive, group or family, short-term or long-term, communication serves as the pathway for its process and procedures.

At its core, communication is the simple exchange of information, but in the context of psychotherapy its most important quality is as a means of persuasion. Persuasive speech is important in many spheres—commerce, politics, religion—and psychotherapeutic persuasion relies on the same principles as do those other disciplines. In those other fields, persuasion is identified as an important skill and is studied and practiced under other names.

- In commerce, salesmanship
- In politics, campaigning
- In religion, preaching

In psychotherapy, however, persuasion has not usually been identified as a necessary and desirable proficiency. Nevertheless, if you intend to be an effective and successful therapist, it will be in your interest to develop the ability to communicate with your patients in a persuasive way.

Key Points

- Communication is a technical skill that is needed to effect persuasive change in therapy.

- Persuasive speech (as distinct from investigative or explanatory discourse) is most effective if it is used sparingly and only at critical moments.

- Metacommunication (indirect commentary) allows the examination of the meaning and motivation of the patient's statements.

- Questions are often more effective than direct statements in investigating and understanding a patient's history.

- Human beings are inherently deceitful, but a therapist must display a credulous and trusting stance, even while maintaining a skeptical and distrustful covert attitude.

- Rhetorical mechanisms can be used to enhance the therapist's ability to convey an idea or persuade a change.

- Modeling is often an effective, nonverbal influence for helpful change.

- Naming, renaming, and reframing are tools that help patients modify their attitude toward their problems.

- Symbolic communication, especially through recounted dreams, may provide unexpected insights into a patient's thoughts and feelings.

CHAPTER
EIGHT

What Is Collaboration?

Coming together is a beginning, staying together is progress, and working together is success.

Henry Ford

Always go to other people's funerals. Otherwise they won't come to yours.

Yogi Berra

Introduction

Most healthcare services are delivered from a caregiver to a suffering recipient. The caregiver prescribes or orders a treatment. The sufferer accepts and assents. In this one-way process, the patient is expected to agree to the treatment decisions of the expert professional, a posture usually termed "compliance."[1] For example, a patient is directed to take all of the tablets of a prescribed drug. (Never mind that only half the prescriptions written are ever filled and that patients often fail to finish all the doses in the bottle.) In this medical model, the patient is passive.

Psychotherapy is different. Most of the time a successful outcome depends on the patient's cooperative engagement with the therapeutic process. After all, only the patient can

* Provide the data necessary to formulate the case. There are no X-rays, biopsies, or laboratory tests.

---

[1]Political correctness now mandates the term "adherence" in place of compliance. Perhaps the next PC step will be to change the heading in the chart from "Doctor's Orders" to "Doctor's Suggestions."

- Describe the perceptions, thoughts, ideas, and feelings on which the therapy operates.
- Change the behavior that is the target of the therapy.

Instead of compliance, successful therapy depends on collaboration, you and the patient working together to realize shared goals, based on the patient's willingness and ability to participate actively in the process. It seems reasonable to expect a successful, voluntary partnership because

- The patient is (frequently) a responsive participant in the therapy;
- (Often) pays "good money" for the service;
- Is (usually) well motivated; and
- Has (presumably) supported the desired outcome and the process needed to reach it.

In spite of these motivating influences, however, in practice the attempt at collaboration is continually undermined by a set of opposing forces. The patient will almost always resist, avoid, manipulate, undermine, or even sabotage the therapy. Much of the work of any therapeutic endeavor is the continuing effort to overcome these reactions and to build up the patient's ability to benefit from the ongoing treatment.

Collaboration is an outgrowth of the therapeutic alliance. That alliance (see Chapter Three[2]) is based on the interaction of your warm, tolerant, empathic concern and the patient's motivation, respect, and hopeful expectation. Its intensity and importance vary. It is usually strongest early on, then gives way to the stresses of the therapy work, and again gains strength as termination approaches (Figure 8–1).

As the alliance confronts the difficult tasks of the methodology—the demands of directive exercises, the dysphoria of successful interpretation, the distress of confronting existential threats—collaboration suffers. No matter how motivated or psychologically minded the patient may be, the ordeal of any therapy and the discomfort of change take their toll. The patient's willing partnership at the outset of therapy, when the alliance is strong, metamorphoses into the stubborn, oppositional, deceptive stance of the middle phases of treatment, when the alliance is most forcefully tested. This chapter reviews several of the challenges to collaborative work and how to deal with them.

---

[2]See pages 83–103.

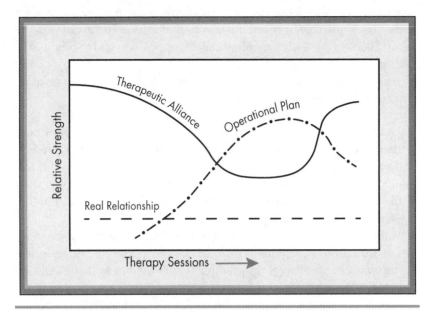

FIGURE 8–1. **Ideal psychotherapy.**

Resistance

Opposed to our effort to make every session count is the apparent contrariness of human nature. When people are told to go right, they will want to turn left, and when asked to go up, they will insist on going down. In therapy work these oppositional and avoidant impulses are called *resistance*. If the purpose of psychotherapy is to bring about a helpful change in behavior, then resistance is, in this context, the opposition to helpful behavioral change. This idea may seem counterintuitive. Why would someone resist a helpful change that is the exact reason for seeking therapy in the first place?

Part of the answer may lie in a fundamental principle of human nature—in fact, of all living things. That principle is *homeostasis*, the tendency to maintain the status quo by acting in opposition to anything that threatens to create an imbalance. Homeostasis is why 95% of people who lose weight regain it within two years. Just as our bodies regulate temperature by shivering or sweating, and even our cells preserve a stable internal environment by shifts in chemical reactions, we attempt to maintain psychic stability by opposing any change with a countervailing force. Even though the patient wants the therapy to work, and you have encouraged this hopeful expectation, each action we make to move the process forward will provoke a counteraction to that effort. The art of psychotherapy lies in your ability to minimize this opposition and to remove the resistance when necessary.

Another reason the patient resists helpful change is the universal instinct of self-protection.

- Unconscious conflict based in early life experiences provokes reactionary defenses designed to minimize its effect on conscious, present-day function. In the earlier example (see Chapter Five[3]) of Phillip's anxiety attack on entering his new office, his response represented his unconscious conflict between the wish and the fear of surpassing (symbolically, displacing) his father.
- Habitual responses to antecedent threats become automatic behaviors that protect the patient from stressful experiences. As an example (see Chapter Two[4]), Elizabeth's habit was not to drive across a bridge. Her avoidance protected her from her learned anxiety response, a compromise between freedom to travel and fear of specific places.

The symptoms for which the patient seeks help represent an unsuccessful effort to deal with threats to psychic stability. Even an unsuccessful effort, however, is preferable to no protection at all. The patient will cling to his or her existing solution and will resist giving it up for whatever untested and uncertain alternative the therapy offers. In fact, the failure of these defenses and habits often is what motivates the patient to seek therapeutic help. Therapy, by challenging these long-standing, ingrained psychological mechanisms, will be experienced not only as a helpful effort but also as a threat. As these "therapy threats" appear, the patient tries to counter them, and the result of the self-protective effort is opposition to therapy solutions.

ABSENCE AS RESISTANCE

Resistance can come in many forms. At its most extreme, it keeps the patient out of your office. The patient shows up late, thus reducing the therapy time, or cancels the appointment, or simply does not appear at all. This effort to reduce exposure to the therapy means the patient feels

---

[3]See page 179.
[4]See page 42.

threatened by whatever is happening in the sessions and chooses this simple, primitive defensive response as a way to avoid the danger.

In this exigent circumstance, you must try to identify, and then reduce or eliminate, the factors that have made the patient feel so menaced as to give up therapy time. The task is more difficult than most attempts to figure out therapy problems because you lack the source of the information, the patient. Thus, the first step is to deal with the patient's absence from the office.

- The correct response to lateness includes an insistence on ending the session at the scheduled time. Extending the time, on the grounds that whatever the patient is avoiding will now emerge, is a mistake. It will reinforce the lateness gambit, since the patient is being rewarded with "extra" time, and it will increase the likelihood of future late arrivals.
- To ignore a cancellation, especially if it is one of a series, is also risky, even though the patient may have what sounds like a perfectly good explanation for it ("I had to take my cat to the vet" or "I forgot I had another appointment"). Even justifications that sound incontrovertible ("My mother had a heart attack") are no guarantee that the patient did not want to miss the session, and the event provided a handy coincidence. The patient who avoids the therapy appointment may take advantage of any convenient reality, but, as in other circumstances, symptomatic behavior is often overdetermined. The reality of the excuse does not negate the way it fits neatly into the patient's need to miss the session. An old therapy maxim puts it: "Reality is the best resistance."
- When the patient fails to cancel and then does not show up for the appointment, the resistance is even more obvious. "I mixed up the time" and "I slept through my alarm" are non-excuse excuses. When you consider that the session is often the patient's most emotionally important event of the week, you can better appreciate the significance of missing it.

Once the patient is again available, you can address the question of what caused the patient to flee the therapy. You can simply ask if the sessions have been upsetting, and many times the patient will be able to tell you why. In other instances, however, the avoidant behavior may be motivated by unconscious, or at best semiconscious, impulses. Although patients may not recognize the motive, they may be able to confirm that missing all or part of the session was accompanied by a sense of relief, of a struggle avoided or of a burden unmet. This recognition then makes the search for the underlying reasons easier. Sometimes, however, the patient will focus only on the conscious, surface reasons until you raise the possibility that other forces may be at work.

INDIRECT RESISTANCE

Most resistance appears in a guise more subtle than not showing up. The patient may employ different strategies designed to avoid a difficult topic or to stay away from a dangerous area of investigation. Each session has only a finite number of minutes. The more of those minutes the patient uses up through resistance behaviors, the fewer are left for active therapy. The patient "chooses" to waste the time in pursuit of a harmless session.

- *Chronicles* are diversionary reports used to fill the time safely. The patient will give a detailed account of occasions and events that occurred since the last meeting, a sort of "how I spent my week" narrative that has no connection with any therapeutic task. Its purpose is to commandeer the time that might otherwise focus on a difficult topic. The chronicle can also be about events that occurred before the last session but that are not related to any of the therapy goals. Again, it simply serves to fill the time and avoid difficult topics. A subtle form of chronicle is the patient's recitation of every adverse event in recent memory because the endless complaints preempt any therapy discussion. To help guide the patient back toward the work of the therapy, you can offer a metacommunication, pointing out the avoidance, or even simply ask, "Why are you telling me about this?"[5] as a way to focus on the chronicle as a problem.
- *Memory lapses*—or, more accurately, memory blocks—are gaps in the patient's recollection of significant portions of history that are connected to the problems the therapy is trying to solve. These are involuntary hiatuses, perhaps due to the mechanism of repression,[6] that only become obvious from the context. As a minor example, if the patient tells you about an earlier incident but cannot recall the

---

[5]Yes, a "why" question (see pages 240–241), but in this case the undertone of disapproval may be helpful.

[6]*Repression* is a psychoanalytic concept, now widely accepted, used to explain how unacceptable or threatening memories and ideas are excluded from conscious recognition.

name of the person involved, the forgotten individual will perhaps be connected with another, embarrassing or frightening event that the patient wishes not to remember. If you can identify the missing material, either from prior knowledge of the patient's history or with the patient's help, you will then have an important focus for future therapy work.

- *Silence* is another form of resistance. If patients come to the session but then have nothing to say, they might as well not be there. Silence can be another form of a late arrival or a missed session. The patient is physically present but therapeutically absent. Two more subtle forms of silence are

  - ➢ *Long pauses.* Patients may speak unusually slowly or allow gaps or pauses to slow their speech production. The effect is to reduce what they will say (literally, the number of words) during the finite period of the session, while they use up the time, avoiding the details of the topic or the topic itself. You can help the patient overcome this type of resistance through a metacommunication. In effect, you choose temporarily to forgo the therapeutic content, which is only dribbling out and not likely to be productive, in favor of a focus on the mechanism—the speech pattern—that is causing the problem.

  - ➢ *Omissions.* Patients who talk around a topic or do not even acknowledge it impose an effective silence. They appear to discuss a subject but in fact are silent about some or all of it. Unless you know, or strongly suspect, what the missing or avoided topic might be, you will have difficulty helping the patient to deal with it. Your best clue to the absence of important material may be your subjective feeling of frustration, your sense that something important is missing, that what you are hearing "doesn't add up." Again, your best response may be a metacommunication in which you interrupt the patient's dilatory or tangential presentation with the observation that you feel there is something missing or that you are not hearing the whole story.

- *Refusal* to discuss a subject is the most overt form of resistance. When patients say, "I can't talk about that" or "It's too hard to talk about," they acknowledge the importance of the subject. A secondary aspect of an outright refusal may be to stir your interest, knowing they have something of importance that will create curiosity and frustration. When this secondary aspect of a communication or other behavior is directed at you, the resistance usually falls into the category of "transference." What the patient means is "I can't talk about that *with*

you" or "It's too hard to talk about *with you*," meaning he or she anticipates you will be critical, judgmental, and disapproving, a clear distortion. The patient's statement about the difficulty of discussing the
topic is a metacommunication on the patient's part. It therefore invites a discussion about the barriers that impede the patient, leaving
the content of the problem for a later point when those barriers have
been removed, or at least lowered.

Although "resistance" and "transference" (discussed in the next section) are terms usually associated with psychodynamic psychotherapy,
such is human nature that they will occur no matter what methodology
you use. Resistance is just as prevalent in behavioral therapies as it is in
psychoanalytic therapies, and requires the same attention.

As an example, suppose you are treating Malcolm, a 42-year-old married man whose fear of flying became a threat when his job description
changed to require monthly business trips involving air travel. Your plan
for the current session involves the identification of triggers related to
his anticipatory anxiety.

Malcolm	I know we're supposed to talk about my problem with flying today, but I don't think I can concentrate on it.
You	Oh?

> *Past experience warns you this digression is not unexpected. The neutral inquiry "Oh?" is preferable to a judgmental "Why not?"*

Malcolm	I had a big fight with my wife this morning, and I can't get my mind off it.
You	Who started it?

> *You suspect it was him, so this question is better than asking what the fight was about.*

Malcolm	I guess I did. She gets upset if I don't pick up after myself, but today I was in a hurry, and I left my clothes and a wet towel on the bathroom floor. She went ballistic.
You	Couldn't you have predicted that?

> *You want to focus on his behavior as a way of uncovering any resistance.*

Malcolm   Sure, if I thought about it, but I was focused on this appointment.

You   Focused how?

Malcolm   Well, I knew we were going to talk about my problem, and I was thinking about what I would say, and I've got that trip at the end of the month, and whether I'd be ready for it.

You   So you're worried about two things. Your apprehension about the treatment itself, and also whether it will work in time.

> *You lay the foundation for interpreting the resistance.*

Malcolm   Yes, talking about flying isn't easy.

You   Do you think you might have provoked the fight today because of those worries?

> *You make the connection for him.*

Malcolm   What? How do you mean?

You   Well, you knew if you left your clothes on the floor your wife would react the way she did. And so far, all we've talked about is that. Because of the fight you avoided the flying problem. I wonder if the fight didn't fit right in with your reluctance to face your anxiety?

> *You offer the interpretation. Using the introductory phrase, "I wonder if..." rather than a bald statement of "fact," that avoids a further transference response.*

Malcolm   You know, it's embarrassing to be afraid to fly. I know it's the safest form of travel. Everybody does it. I feel like a coward.

> *Although he does not concede the point, he brings up a new issue and returns to the therapy plan.*

Resistance can appear in many forms, and these few examples by no means cover its protean nature. Whenever the progress of a therapy slows or stops, you can be sure your patient is having difficulty with the task at hand and, consciously or unconsciously, is doing something to avoid it. In this general sense, any behavior on the patient's part that is inconsistent with the treatment contract, or that impedes the therapeutic work, is resistance. Because resistance is ubiquitous, dealing with it could take up most (or in some therapies, like psychoanalysis, all) of every session. To avoid this preoccupation, keep in mind the following rule: *Deal with resistance only when you have no other way of making progress in the therapy.*

This stricture means, for instance, that you should not interpret the first missed session or late arrival or the second or even the third. Wait and see if you can make progress with the time available. Only when you conclude that you cannot should you ask the patient to consider the way the behavior impacts the agreed-on task. As another example of this restraint, you might ignore a short chronicle, perhaps in the first few minutes of the session, as the patient's way of easing into the therapeutic work. Only when the chronicle threatens to take too much time is it worth using even more time to deal with it.

In planning the treatment, you have usually set some number of goals, perhaps only two or as many as four. At any given moment, the therapy should be moving toward one of those objectives (working toward more than one at a time is usually not productive), and the difficulty you encounter may be limited to just the current task. Perhaps you can shift focus to another goal without encountering the same degree of resistance, particularly if the alternative goal requires a different method of therapy. For example, if your treatment plan for Malcolm included both a behavioral strategy to deal with the phobia and a second goal of an improved marital relationship, using a transactional approach, you could continue the session with work on the marital problem. The overriding consideration, then, is to make progress as long as possible and only pause to deal with resistance when it is not.

Transference

Conscious or unconscious avoidance occurs when the therapeutic subject matter seems too anxiety-provoking or embarrassing or connected with guilty or shameful feelings. Since this type of evasion depends in large part on how the patient expects you to respond, it often signals a transference problem. The patient anticipates condemnation, condescension, criticism, or some other negative response from you. Presumably, you have done nothing to justify these negative expectations:

- In pursuit of a strong therapeutic alliance, you have been nonjudgmental and committed to unconditional positive regard.
- You have not treated any previous revelations with other than acceptance and an interest in understanding them.

Since you are not the source of the patient's apprehensions, then they must be self-generated and must arise from the patient's experience with somebody from the past. This earlier experience generates an attitude that is now *transferred* to you. At least, that is your argument when you invite the patient to step back from the reaction and to explore who among the people from earlier in life might have been the author of the feelings they have mistakenly ascribed to you. At times, of course, you have a strong suspicion, based on the patient's history, who that someone might be, and you can simply ask whether that is the source of the feeling toward you.

It is often useful, as you try to establish that some past figure of authority or importance, and not you, is the real source of their expectation, to ask patients to identify any specifics about you or your past behavior that would support their judgment. Often the best way to explore the issue is simply to ask, "What is the evidence for it?" There may be none, in which case it is easy to redirect the patient's attention to whomever in the past fits the picture they mistakenly had of you. If the patient can cite some observations that underlie the role you are supposed to play—and if none of the instances is accurate—you can review each of them and correct the impression it may have made. For example, if a patient says, "You laughed when I told you I couldn't find my car," you can remind him that you only laughed (with him) after you confessed that the same thing happened to you.

The clarity of the distinction you want the patient to make, however, rests on your innocence of any of the behavior of which you stand accused. If the patient claims you have actually demonstrated the attitude that justifies the accusation, your alleged prior conduct, if true, will undercut your invitation to examine the problem as a transference reaction.

- You may, in fact, have exhibited the sentiments the patient now remembers. In that case, the therapy challenge is to distinguish that past event from the present circumstances. This task is not always easy, but it can be done if you can evince sufficient evidence of the historical basis for the patient's current feelings; if, for example, you can juxtapose the rage shown by the patient's father with the mild annoyance you might have displayed previously, or if you can show that your trivial criticism pales before the outright condemnation the patient experienced with a grade-school teacher. In these instances, you hope to contrast the insignificance of some previous display of yours with the immensity of the hurt the patient suffered in the past. In other words, the misrepresentation is the magnitude of the earlier problem contrasted with your present behavior. Use that difference to show that, in fact, the patient's impression of you is actually a transference distortion.

- The patient's appraisal of your past behavior may, in itself, represent a transference reaction. In other words, the patient may remember and interpret your past behavior as *earlier* transference feelings that were concealed or missed. In that case, your task becomes somewhat easier, since you can now point out that both instances are misrepresentations of your actual behavior and are based on past experience with someone else. Here the transference distortion appears as the patient's hypersensitivity through which your actions have been filtered.

Unlike the case with ordinary resistance, for which you defer action until you cannot make further progress, the patient's overt transference toward you usually requires immediate intervention. Even if only a hint of the attitude emerges, it may impact the entire therapy effort. If the patient sees you as condescending, critical, authoritarian, punitive, or in any otherwise distorted posture, that problem requires whatever time is needed to reverse it. The therapeutic alliance itself is under attack, and the rupture must be repaired before the patient can regain the trust and confidence needed for therapy to progress.

To review the process, you may need some or all of the following steps:

- Start by attempting to get a full picture of what is involved in the transferred attitude. How does the description fit somebody from the patient's past? You may require additional history to make that connection.
- Ask the patient (if you do not already know) to think of whose past treatment parallels the way the patient thinks you are behaving now.
- Next, ask the patient to point out whatever he or she believes the evidence is that you actually are the way the patient thinks you are. If possible, point out the contrary evidence from your past and current behavior toward the patient.

- If you can make the connection between past and present, especially when you have established that the person in question is not you, the patient will often be able to correct the distortion and therapy can move forward.

Consider the following example. Your patient, Carol, is a 30-year-old woman raised by a critical and demanding mother. You suspect, from previous discussions, that Carol's mother was an insecure woman who was jealous of any attention Carol's father paid to his daughter.

Carol	I'm really upset by something you said last time.
You	What was it?
Carol	I told you that I received a good performance review at work, the best I ever got, and you just blew it off. *From your history you already recognize that she thinks you are like her mother (and perhaps others in her experience.)*
You	How did you hope I'd take the news? *You ask for more data.*
Carol	Well, I didn't expect a standing ovation, but some recognition would have been nice.
You	Hmm. How would you have felt if I'd stood up and applauded? *You take her exaggeration literally in order to reflect its oddity, a rhetorical device.*
Carol	(*thinks for a moment*) Like you were making fun of me.
You	So does that mean that even a positive reaction feels like a criticism to you? *You highlight a further anomaly in her response to your neutral behavior.*
Carol	Maybe.
You	That's what your mother was like, wasn't it? Nothing you ever did was good enough. *You make an interpretive connection.*

Carol   Everything I did was wrong.

You   But you kept hoping she would give you some rec-
             ognition.

                         You underline the transference feeling.

Carol   Yes.

You   And now you're looking for the same appreciation
             from me.

                         At this point you have made the con-
                         nection and can explore the problem
                         with her mother further.

Transference issues are more likely to occur, or to occur more quickly, in proportion to the opacity of the therapist, or, in other words, how much of yourself you have revealed to the patient. Self-disclosure, however, always requires careful judgment: too little will provoke inappropriate emotion, but too much will risk disrespect. Or, from another one of Aesop's fables, "familiarity breeds contempt."

The less the patient knows about you, and the more blanks there are in your persona, the easier it is for the patient to fill those blanks with feelings and perceptions from the patient's past. The desire to minimize transference development, however, should not lure you into revealing more personal information than might otherwise be appropriate. Transference, at least to some degree, is inevitable in any extended therapy, and it can be successfully defused without a prolonged disruption of therapeutic progress. An overly open and revealing therapist, like the idol with feet of clay, risks a permanent loss of status. One important facet of the role of healer (a key feature of the therapeutic alliance) is the implied social standing and power that society grants to the role. Part of that power is the mystery inherent in the healer's role. Once that mystery evaporates and the healer's status fades, it may never be regained.

The degree to which a therapist remains an unknown and mysterious person is usually referred to as the "blank screen" effect—the idea being that the patient projects onto the "screen" whatever unresolved or troublesome relationships create unconscious pressure for expression. The "blank screen" metaphor is somewhat overstated, however, because transference distortions occur even when the other person is well known and has a long personal history with the patient. In marriages, for example, despite the intimate relationship and years of togetherness, these distortions can create persistent misunderstandings and strains.

- A woman whose parents were sneaky and conniving, for example, may view her husband with unwarranted suspicion.
- A man whose mother was depressed and withholding might feel chronically unloved by his devoted wife.

In the same way, even if you are more open and revealing about personal matters you may still provoke transference reactions as the therapy becomes more intense. Moreover, the more the patient knows about you, the harder it may be to draw a distinction between yourself and the person from the past with whom you are being confused.

Countertransference

When you project your own unresolved past problems onto the patient, instead of transference it is called *countertransference*, although in fact the process is exactly the same. The distortion that arises from your confusion of the patient's behavior with some past experience of your own can be just as problematic for the therapy as when the patient misjudges you. The important distinction, however, is that you have no one else to recognize the problem (with the possible exception of a supervisor) and must rely on your own efforts. Most of the time you must depend on a high index of suspicion and your observing ego to help you flag, and quickly deal with, those feelings.

- One exercise that can be helpful in picking up your countertransference feelings is to ask yourself, perhaps each morning before you start to meet patients, which one you *least* want to see that day. Then ask yourself why that is true.
  - ➢ Does the patient "push the wrong buttons"?
  - ➢ Who else does that to you?
  - ➢ What exactly do you dislike about that person?
  - ➢ Who else have you known with those same characteristics?
- You should also ask yourself which patient you most want to see that day. Countertransference feelings, like transference feelings, can be positive as well as negative, and the patient you most want to see may be one that excites your rescue fantasies or some other inappropriate interest.

This kind of self-examination may flag a countertransference problem before it becomes a hindrance to therapy with that patient.

For example, suppose the patient you least want to see is a man a few years younger than you, and you realize that you have found him more and more annoying over the course of several therapy sessions. As you think back on his behavior, you realize that he tends to challenge everything you say and is almost disrespectful in his arrogant posture of knowing all the answers. With reflection you recognize that he reminds you of your younger brother, the little brat you resented, especially when he was more successful in vying for your parents' attention. Once you identify that your reaction to your annoying patient is a holdover from the sibling rivalry of your childhood, it should be easier to deal with your patient. Perhaps his annoying behavior reflects his own unresolved feelings with an older sibling or his need to appear competent even when he feels frightened inside. By shifting your attention away from your own feelings you may be in a better position to understand the patient's and to help him deal with them.

Provoked Emotion: The Geiger Counter Effect

In contrast to countertransference reactions, your feelings toward a patient may reflect the patient's subliminal efforts to stimulate a particular response, efforts that grow out of his or her own problems and not yours. In other words, your attitude toward a patient sometimes originates, not in your own unresolved past conflicts, but in the patient's attitudes and responses to you. The specific determinants of your reaction may be easily identifiable in the ongoing behavior of the patient or may be only a subtle influence hard to immediately recognize. The behavior may be overt, as when a patient speaks in a threatening tone of voice, or covert, as when you feel threatened but do not immediately know why. The patient may be only partially aware of the provocation or its source may be unconscious. Your emotional response to the patient might appear to be unrelated to the content of the session, whatever topic is under discussion at that moment.

To mention a few examples, you might feel

- Frustrated.
- Angry.
- Anxious.
- Fearful.
- Stimulated.
- Bored.

Alertness to these provoked emotions is often an early indication of a transference stirring within the patient or may represent a latent character trait or other symptomatic behavior. A prompt awareness can prevent a more difficult situation that would develop later if the transference or trait or behavior is ignored. In this respect you should function like a therapeutic Geiger counter, picking up emotional radiation instead of gamma rays. If you feel

- Frustrated, then the patient is attempting to frustrate you.
- Angry, then the patient is trying to provoke your anger.
- Anxious, then the patient wishes to unsettle you.
- Fearful, then the patient wants to intimidate you.
- Stimulated, then the patient is flirting with you or trying to provoke a sexual response.
- Bored, then the patient is avoiding something important by droning on about irrelevant or trivial matters.

In order to understand what is meant by these covert communications, you must first ask yourself, "Why does this patient want me to feel this way?" The answer may be obvious, but often the solution requires a period of active exploration and interpretation. The sequence of events would be to

- Recognize the feeling and attitude change, using your observing ego function, as discussed in the chapter on the initial evaluation and elsewhere.
- Establish that it does not represent your internal response (as in the usual countertransference) through self-examination.
- Identify the phenomenon to the patient, including that it is something the patient has evoked.
- Ask the patient to confirm or deny it, and
    - ➤ If confirmed, explore the basis for the patient's behavior.
    - ➤ If denied, suggest you and the patient try to determine why it occurred.

These provoked responses may primarily be the result of the patient's nonverbal influences on you and are not necessarily revealed by the content of the patient's verbal production. Understanding their source requires an appreciation not only of the immediate context but also of the historical and emotional background. For example, the covertly seductive patient may have a history of abuse and need to test whether you will take advantage of the asymmetrical relationship in the way an earlier abuser did.

For another example, here is the beginning of a session with Blake, a 23-year-old college senior, whose roommate, Jim, killed himself while at home during the winter vacation break. In the last session, Blake's verbal production slowed, and he did not speak for the last ten minutes. You know from your evaluation that Blake has a normal mental status, an above-average IQ, and no evidence of a psychosis.

You	How are you today?
Blake	I've been…I don't…the last time you said…
You	(*when he does not continue*) I said what?
Blake	You said…I was wondering…I thought…I don't know…
You	Do you realize you haven't completed a single sentence this morning?
	At this point you feel impatient and are beginning to get angry.
Blake	I guess…but what if I…I don't want to…
You	What's going on?
	Your anger grows and you feel hard pressed to keep the irritation out of your voice.
Blake	Jim killed himself…
You	Yes, I know. That's why we're meeting. What about Jim?
	You wonder if you can ask him to leave and come back when he is ready to talk.
Blake	He killed himself…He…I…
	You have no reason to think Blake's mental status has deteriorated to the point where he cannot complete a sentence. Has he suddenly developed thought blocking, a symptom of schizophrenia? Not likely. Could he be speaking in these

tantalizing phrases to provoke the very impatience and anger you feel toward him? You think back to the previous session. What was happening just before he shut down and ended the session in silence? You recall he was ruminating about whether he was responsible for Jim's suicide and whether he could have, or should have, done something to stop it.

You Blake, you told me last week you felt you were at fault somehow about Jim's decision to end his life. Is that what's on your mind today?

Blake You didn't say anything when I told you that. It's like you agreed with me, but you didn't want me to know it. I thought about it all week. You must really dislike me. The least you can do is talk about it.
    Suddenly, he begins to speak again, suggesting you have tapped into the motive for his earlier, halting speech.

You I guess I made you angry when I didn't comment on what you were feeling.
    You acknowledge his feelings.

Blake It's like you didn't care.
    Without meaning to, your silence in the prior session damaged the therapeutic alliance and the result was this piece of acting-out behavior.

You And now you're doing the same thing to me. Starting a sentence and letting me wonder about what you're thinking. Giving me little hints and never telling me your whole thought. A taste of my own medicine. Showing me what it feels like.
    Now that Blake is talking and you seem to have identified the reason he made you angry, you and he can address his grievance.

Splitting

A special instance of provoked emotion is splitting. In Chapter Four,[7] I mentioned it as a phenomenon to look for in the initial interview. To recap: splitting is a reflection of all-or-nothing thinking, something that is judged as all good or all bad, rather than the mixture of qualities that is usually the case. Splitting is especially troublesome when the patient portrays someone in terms that depict that individual as all bad (an evil person who has disadvantaged, neglected, or damaged the patient) or all good (someone who—often with the implication of "unlike you"—was a benign, nurturing, helpful saint). In this context, splitting should be suspected when the patient describes someone to you in a way that provokes your strong emotional response either for or against a person you do not know.

For example, a patient may describe a previous therapist in terms that lead you to conclude that the other therapist mistreated your patient or neglected some obvious problem. You may even find yourself concluding that your patient was a victim of malpractice. The sense of outrage you feel should act as a red flag and alert you that the patient has provoked your response by a selective or possibly false account. What you have heard might even be true or have at least a kernel of truth, but it almost certainly is not the full story. It could represent a falsification of memory or a transference distortion. Even if it was true, the fact that you have been stirred up emotionally means you are not able to deal with the patient's account in a dispassionate and helpful manner. The issue has gone from a therapy topic to a potential cause of action. The better response, once you have recognized that your reaction has been provoked, is to consider what motive—conscious or unconscious—your patient may have in exciting you that way. Does the patient

- Benefit from your thinking of her or him as a victim?
- Seek the gratification of having you leap to his or her defense?
- Want to provoke your anger at the other person as a way of controlling you?
- Wish to undermine your neutral therapist's stance in order to prove you really care?

This type of distortion can create real problems for the therapy and, in fact, for you personally. If, for instance, you accept the patient's presenta-

---

[7]See page 118.

tion as a helpless victim you might underestimate or miss altogether the patient's need to adopt such a role. If you believe (in the above example) that another therapist has mistreated your patient, you may act toward that therapist in ways that damage your professional standing.

Splitting is common in individual therapy[8] because, almost always, the patient is your only source of information. As an analogy, consider how a country with a dictatorship that controls its media will mislead the population in order to better control it. State-controlled Russian news sources, for instance, selectively provide only unfavorable news about the West and, often, falsely positive news about Russia's rulers. No wonder the Russian people distrust other nations and hugely approve of their leaders. The patient's inclination to provide a distorted version of someone unknown to you usually reflects their general "pathology," however, and is not a malicious effort to manipulate you. Rather, it often reveals needs and motives of which the patient is unaware. It then becomes a therapeutic task to explore, understand, and possibly correct these covert tendencies.

Splitting may involve all kinds of people from the patient's current or past life, but most often, and most importantly, it involves close and meaningful relationships. The distorted picture of family members, romantic partners, friends, and business associates will often mirror the same problems for which the patient sought treatment. Your sensitivity to the provoked responses that signal these distortions will allow you to identify and help to correct the problems on which they are based. This interaction with the patient is where the skeptical side of your observing ego can save you from manipulation to your and the patient's detriment. When you feel yourself stirred emotionally by the patient's description of someone, always ask yourself, "Is this really true?" If the answer is "Maybe not," and what you hear is only the patient's version of that person, splitting may be the reason.

Boundary Violations

Part of the real relationship (see Chapter Three[9]) is a group of "rules" that together form the boundaries of the therapist-patient association. These rules are not only unwritten, they are usually unspoken and are assumed to be understood. Among these rules:

---

[8]Even though splitting is closely associated with borderline personality disorder, it is a common and widespread feature of many patient presentations.
[9]See pages 75–83.

- The length (in minutes) of the scheduled sessions is predetermined and fixed.
- Patient-therapist interaction should occur only in a session.
- The therapy service is rendered in return for a specified payment.
- Payment is expected at time of service (or as billed on a regular schedule).
- The patient-therapist association is a professional relationship, not a personal one.
- The therapist's personal (extra-professional) life is private.
- Only the therapist can change the rules.

These conditions (and sometimes others) form a social contract between the two parties. Even if they are never discussed, the majority of patients will have no difficulty with them and will honor the implied contract. Any breach will therefore stand out in conspicuous contrast to business-as-usual, and it should be dealt with swiftly and decisively. When a boundary violation is ignored, or allowed to "rewrite" the terms of agreement, the result will not only damage the therapy but it will place you under undue stress.

Boundary violations can take many forms and are sometimes subtle and easy to miss (Table 8–1). Some of the more obvious violations occur when patients

- Attempt to overstay their time. They may keep talking after you have said the session is over or linger at the door while adding "Just one more thing…"
- Come to the office without an appointment or "accidently" meet you outside of the office.
- Contact you by telephone (or email or text) about issues that should be discussed in session. Sometimes these contacts are disguised as "emergencies" when they are not life-threatening situations.
- Skip or delay payments or otherwise fail to render their portion of the fee.
- Make inappropriate inquiries and comments about personal aspects of your life, either in the session or through online research. At its extreme, a patient may physically stalk you.
- Vie for control of the process through attempts to unilaterally change the "rules" of the social contract. For example, a patient who walks in and sits in your chair.

These boundary violations can be considered severe *symptomatic acts*; that is, they are behavioral expressions of internal conflicts and traits. An

TABLE 8–1. Boundary violations

Boundary	Characteristics	Violation example: patient will
Session	Length	Overstay time
Session	Location	Waylay therapist away from office
Payment	Amount	Fail to pay or only make partial payment
Payment	When due	Delay or miss payments
Privacy	Personal	Make inappropriate inquiries or comments
Privacy	Physical	Do online research about therapist, stalk therapist
Control	Rules	Make unilateral revisions to social contract

example of an ordinary symptomatic act: a man who trips at the door every time he enters the office conveys the message, "I'm stumbling through life." This common type of symptomatic behavior, one that does not disrupt the social contract, can be treated as simply another communication by the patient and, as such, can be useful in the therapy. A true boundary violation, however, threatens the therapy and must first be confronted and blocked before making any attempt to use it.

Patients with borderline personality disorder, for example, will often make attempts to reach you between appointments, perhaps with the announcement that they feel like hurting themselves. If you accept this "emergency" and provide, essentially, an extra session on the telephone (or even more time than in a face-to-face session), the patient will be likely to call again…and again and again and again. These telephone sessions will not make the patient any less desperate and will not advance the treatment plan. The necessary response is to direct the patient to the emergency room or offer to call the police and an ambulance, or whatever action is needed to reject the attempt to manipulate the contract. You can then refuse to engage in a long telephone discussion and suggest it will be important to discuss the behavior at the next regular session. Initially, this effort may simply increase the emotional blackmail ("I'll kill myself, and it'll be all your fault."), but each escalation must be blocked as well.

Whatever the manifestation of a boundary violation—refusal to leave the office, nonpayment of fees, and so forth—the response should be the same: block first, analyze second. If the behavior persists and the boundary cannot be reestablished, the result may be an early termination and referral elsewhere.

Timing of Interventions

When you formulate a case you begin to reach conclusions, constructed at first as merely hypotheses but later confirmed or modified by the clinical evidence. Those conclusions will point to areas of behavior that are dysfunctional and counterproductive and that need to change if therapy is to make progress. If you could only tell the patient, at the end of the initial interview, "Here's what you need to do," and the patient would do it! Alas, that's not the way it works.

Freud discovered this flaw early on when he thought he had only to reveal to patients (after two or three weeks) the unconscious conflicts that underlay their symptoms and they would be cured. When "making the unconscious conscious" failed to work, his analyses went from weeks to months to (sometimes) years. So, today, even though early on you may have the answers to your patients' difficulties, the key to effective therapy is the timing of your interventions.

This requirement is most clearly seen in psychodynamic psychotherapy, where the intervention is in the form of an interpretation. An interpretation is most easily accepted if it is offered when the patient is just on the verge of making the discovery on his or her own. Your job is then to put into words an idea the patient already has vaguely in mind and therefore will "feel" is right. In psychodynamic work this principle is called "staying on the surface" and is usually coupled with the advice, "Begin where the patient is at."

The same principle of timing applies to other methodologies as well. You never want to lead the patient into areas he or she is not prepared to go. In directive therapies, this idea often means you need to spend sufficient time educating, explaining, and preparing patients before you ever ask, or direct, them to undergo whatever exercise you think will help. The same approach holds true for the experiential therapies as well.

To develop this sense of timing you can rely on your empathic connection with your patients to give you a sense of whether they are ready for the next step or need more preparatory work. Accumulated experience with the timing of interventions and their result will help you become more and more successful in making these judgments.

As examples of timing we can look again at two of the cases discussed earlier.

- Elizabeth's bridge phobia (see Chapter Two[10]) required a period of preparation in which she visualized, at home, driving over the bridge. In the interval between sessions this exercise reduced her anxiety from 85 out of 100 to only 30. She could then drive over the bridge with you beside her. If you had asked her to drive over the bridge in the first session, when her anxiety at merely visualizing the trip was still quite high, she would not have agreed or been able to complete the trip if she had tried.
- The formulation for Phillip (see Chapter Five[11]), who had a panic attack on entering his office as a new vice president, suggested that his anxiety originated in an unresolved, unconscious conflict with his recently deceased father. You would need a number of exploratory sessions before you could confront him with this interpretation. If you had immediately said to him, "You panicked because when you outdid your father, you were frightened that he would retaliate from beyond the grave," he might have laughed it off, agreed on an intellectual level, or even become more anxious. The premature interpretation would have been useless, however, in helping him to resolve his problem.

Management of Defenses

You will often need to confront and challenge your patients on what you have identified as their major psychological defense mechanisms. You do this in the belief (and the hope) that you will remove barriers to change and allow them to adopt more successful behaviors. For example, you may

- Ask a phobic patient to give up the avoidance and to enter the anxiety-provoking environment.
- Challenge the emotional isolation of an obsessional patient to reduce the rigidity of a habit.
- Highlight the logical inconsistency of a negative overgeneralization in order to diminish automatic thoughts.

---

[10]See page 42.
[11]See page 179.

In each case, you act on two assumptions:

1. The patient is psychologically strong enough to withstand the consequences of removing a protective defense.
2. The discarded defense will be replaced with more functional and adaptive behavior.

The patients about whom you can have the greater confidence that these assumptions are correct are, in fact, those patients who are psychologically stronger and mentally healthier. In Chapter Four[12] I described these patients as being toward the high-functioning end of a suitability continuum.

Sometimes, however, even a high-functioning patient may struggle with impenetrable defenses. As an example: I once asked a young professional who had difficulty with assertiveness to undertake one "aggressive action" before the next session. I imagined that he would engage in an argument or insist on his rights. When he returned, he reported that he had succeeded. "Someone offered me a stick of gum," he said, "and I took it." For this man, accepting a trivial gift was an act of aggression.

The situation is quite different, however, with patients who are at the lower-functioning end of the suitability spectrum. Their defenses are already shaky and only partially successful. Dysphoric emotions may threaten to overwhelm them, diminishing even further their ability to function. Primitive conflicts and problems with reality-based thinking may be barely restrained. In short, a successful challenge to the defenses of these patients could result in a significant deterioration of their mental health.

Your approach to these patients, then, should be to strengthen their existing defenses, even at the risk of sacrificing possible overall improvement, at least until such time as you judge them to be more resilient and psychologically stronger. Instead of offering an interpretation that uncovers conflict and reveals hidden motivation, you can support the denial or displacement or whatever you think is holding the dysfunction in check.

Suppose, for example, your patient is a man who recently recovered from a psychotic decompensation but who now appears stable on medication and in a less stressful environment. During the session, he says, "I had a dream last night that my father died and my mother wanted me to take over his business." This manifest dream might lead you, with

---

[12]See pages 119–120.

another and healthier patient, into a useful discussion of oedipal issues. With your current patient, however, the direct emergence of early developmental material could prove, to say the least, unsettling. Instead of discussing his "wish" for his father's death, you could say to him that the dream shows his mother's appreciation for his competence and reliability. This strengthening effort is usually referred to as "interpreting upward." It means you ignore the underlying conflict and emphasize the positive, contemporary and supportive elements of the patient's behavior. You can also strengthen shaky defenses by more direct means. You can suggest helpful strategies to deal with stress or, in a case management approach, you can try to engineer changes that reduce environmental stresses in the patient's life.

For those patients in the midrange of the suitability continuum—and they will usually be the majority—your stance on dealing with defenses must strike a balance between early confrontation and strengthening defenses. This balance often means a gradual chipping away at the patient's dysfunctional behavioral strategies. Starting with a gentle challenge on the most obvious manifestations, you persist, bit by bit, until you have revealed the entire problem. An analogy would be the work of an archeologist, carefully removing layer after layer until the whole artifact is uncovered and can be removed.

Advice

In a comedy skit first aired in 1960 when psychoanalysis was a dominant influence, an interviewer (Carl Reiner) asks a "famous psychiatrist" (Mel Brooks) to tell him about one of his successful cases. To paraphrase: Brooks says he cured a young woman who had been isolated in her house, doing nothing all day but tearing up pieces of paper. Years of analysis had failed to help her.

> REINER: That's amazing! Nobody could help her, but you did? How did you do it?
> BROOKS: Well, I went to her, and I said, "Don't tear paper. You're a nice young woman. Go out and meet people, go to a party, a social function, but just don't tear paper!"
> REINER (*admiringly*): That's it? That did it? She was cured?
> BROOKS: She never tore paper again.

The "Don't Tear Paper" school of psychotherapy operates on the principle that simple advice will empower behavior change. If only! In reality, if patients' problems merely required straightforward advice they would not need you. Patients have already heard an unhelpful and ineffective abundance of suggestions and recommendations before they ever get to you. The temptation to substitute advice for the hard work of therapy, however, is insidious and pervasive. At times, the solution to a patient's problem seems so obvious that you might find yourself offering the answer, even if the patient has not asked for it. Bear in mind, however, that

- The patient almost always knows what should be done but is unable to do it.
- Family, friends, blogs, television therapists, and multiple other sources have often already provided advice, along with exhortations, pleas, and other manipulations, all to no avail.
- Your "advice" can be misinterpreted as an order, a coercion, or the imposition of your will on the patient, with the predictable responses of resentment, defiance, false agreement, or the provocation of (perhaps justifiable) transference feelings.
- Even when your behavioral advice is useful and the patient follows it successfully, the benefit is limited and may not help the patient function with an independent judgment. Remember the saying "Give a man a fish and you feed him a meal. Teach him to fish and you feed him for a lifetime."

In general, the best advice about giving advice is "Don't do it."

Occasionally, however, circumstances will arise when it is actually helpful to give advice. Consider the following "analyst joke": A patient tells his analyst he feels suicidal and thinks he should get up off the couch and jump out the window.

ANALYST: Hmmm…
PATIENT (*standing up*): All right, I'll do it.
ANALYST: Hmmm…
PATIENT (*goes to window and raises the sash*): I'm going to jump.
ANALYST: Hmmm…
PATIENT: Here I go. (*Jumps.*)
ANALYST (*goes to window and looks down*): Hmmm…

Clearly, the advice needed is "Don't jump," and any situation of risk or danger requires active intervention, and Advice with a capital A. In less dire circumstances, advice may be helpful when

- You have important information that the patient lacks. For example, if the patient has been given a medication that you know will adversely react with a drug already prescribed.

- The patient, through ignorance or naiveté, contemplates a decision you know will be a serious, even catastrophic, mistake. For example, a patient who wants to propose marriage to someone after only three dates.
- You have expert knowledge the patient is not likely to find elsewhere. For example, if the patient is unaware of a government benefit you know they will be eligible to receive.

Perhaps other special circumstances will arise where your advice can be helpful, but, as the above examples suggest, these should be concrete practical situations. When you are dealing with the patient's emotional or psychological problems, advice is almost never an effective intervention.

Support

Supportive psychotherapy is a widely used term that encompasses a variety of interventions and techniques borrowed from other, more clearly defined methodologies. It is often applied to two starkly contrasting types of patient:

1. Essentially healthy individuals temporarily overwhelmed by stressful circumstances. This group of patients usually falls within the "situational" classification described in Chapter Five[13] as a formulation category. The plan with these individuals is to "support" their intrinsic coping abilities to allow them spontaneously to heal and recover their previous level of function.
2. Severely and chronically ill individuals who are judged able to improve with "support" but who are expected, by reason of their diagnosis, to remain ill and never to recover fully from their illness.

In both instances, however, the patient will still benefit from a treatment plan that outlines the desired result, the goals that will achieve it, and the strategies needed to reach those objectives.

In a broader sense, however, the term "supportive," when used to describe a proposed treatment plan, is meaningless:

- All therapies are supportive because the healing forces of the therapeutic alliance and the active treatment plan are present in any effective modality.

---

[13]See pages 170–173.

- No strategies or techniques are specific to "supportive therapy." All of its interventions and approaches have been developed under the aegis of other methodologies and include elements of expressive, directive, and experiential therapies.

Seen in this framework, supportive therapy is simply another name for an eclectic psychotherapy.

A more serious problem with the idea of "support" arises when it becomes the fallback strategy in a therapy effort that has reached an impasse or has failed to achieve a good outcome. As outlined in Chapter Six,[14] the source of this failure is often an incomplete or missing treatment plan. As a result of the impasse:

- You and the patient continue to meet without any further improvement in the patient's problems.
- The therapy is no longer focused on reaching its treatment goals.
- The relationship between you and the patient remains positive, and both of you are reluctant to give it up.
- Sessions begin to revolve about day-to-day problems for which you can make "helpful comments" or even give advice (see above) and opportunities for the patient to "vent" feelings for which you simply lend a sympathetic ear.
- Since neither of you any longer expects to reach a specified outcome, therapy can continue for as long as time and money are available: an interminable treatment.

Rather than settle for a "supportive" solution to a treatment that is stalled and unproductive, the better response is to

- Find the reason for the impasse: problems with the plan or with the treatment contract; therapy problems like resistance and transference.
- Reassess the patient and, if necessary, make a new, overt plan.

Final Thoughts

The relatively simple concepts described in this chapter (see Table 8–2, page 290, for summary) have wide applicability since they address issues that will occur in many therapies, regardless of the modality and

---

[14]See pages 214–215.

methods employed. Although some of them are "claimed" by a particular methodology—the concept of "transference" by the psychodynamic school, for instance—in fact, the problems with which they deal are more a product of the general process of therapy than of the more limited area encompassed by a specific method.

To put this idea more clearly: they fall within the compass of the therapeutic alliance. To the extent that the alliance relies on a progressive, empathic, and caring relationship,

- The multiple determinants of resistance will run counter to the overt agreement for a collaborative effort to solve the patient's problems.
- The emergence of transference and countertransference feelings will undermine the strength of the relationship.
- Boundary violations will challenge, and sometimes break, the basic agreement needed to conduct therapy in a protected and safe environment.
- Mistimed interventions and mismanaged handling of defenses will weaken the bonds of trust and reliability.
- The inappropriate use of advice and the surrender to "supportive" therapy will invalidate the working basis for the common purposes agreed on by both participants.

The therapeutic alliance is at its core a collaborative partnership between you and the patient, but its strength fluctuates over the course of therapy as the pursuit of the agreed-upon goals clashes with the reality of the difficulty of change. The strains may diminish the intensity of the patient's commitment and sometimes temporarily rupture it. An awareness of the specific dynamics behind the strains will allow you to deal with them earlier and more successfully.

Key Points

- Successful therapy outcomes depend on the combined efforts of both you and the patient.
- This partnership is a practical manifestation of the therapeutic alliance.
- The collaborative effort provokes counterforces that threaten its success.
- Recognition of these counterforces allows early and effective corrections that facilitate good treatment outcomes.

- Resistance appears in all therapeutic modalities and includes the special cases of transference and countertransference.

- Patients sometimes undermine the partnership by provoking you or violating the terms of the therapy agreement.

- Progress is enhanced by the proper timing of interventions and the careful management of defenses.

- Inappropriate use of advice and using "support" as a substitute for overcoming treatment impasses will undermine treatment outcomes.

TABLE 8–2. Challenges to collaboration

Type of challenge	Examples
Overt resistance	Missed session, lateness, cancelled session
Covert resistance	Chronicles, silence, memory lapse, refusal to discuss
Transference	Distorted conclusion about your motives
Countertransference	Distorted conclusion about the patient's motives
Provoked emotion	Your unexplained feelings of frustration, anxiety, and so forth; splitting
Boundary violations	Patients who resist the end of sessions
Timing of interventions	Premature interpretation
Management of defenses	"Upward" interpretation for fragile patient
Advice	Direct suggestions about symptomatic behavior
Support	Abandonment of treatment goals after treatment impasse

CHAPTER
NINE

What Is an Autodidact?

Reading maketh a full man, conference a
ready man, and writing an exact man.

Francis Bacon

If you ask me anything I don't know, I'm not
going to answer.

Yogi Berra

Introduction

Previous chapters have focused on generic psychotherapy issues, but
now we turn to specific psychotherapies, or, rather, to how to become
skilled in them after you have completed your training.

Formal education in any of the mental health specialties will leave
most prospective therapists feeling underprepared in psychotherapy.
Current training programs divide the educational time among several
areas, including inpatient care, psychopharmacology, diagnostic evaluation, basic sciences, and research. Psychotherapy may not be taught as
a formal subject, particularly as its instruction relies on a kind of appren-
tice system in which the trainee is assigned therapy cases under the tu-
telage of a supervisor. The number of cases that can be followed in this
system is limited. Didactic preparation is less available and may rely too
much on a "cookbook" approach. These limitations mean that for most
people interested in a full therapy practice (or even part-time work), after leaving the training program, you are on your own.

An autodidact is a self-educated person, and history records many
famous examples. Benjamin Franklin, Charles Darwin, Leonardo da Vinci,
Ernest Hemingway, and Frank Lloyd Wright were all autodidacts. Ther-

apists who wish to improve and expand their skills must be autodidacts by necessity. Not only is formal coursework a rare commodity after training ends, but even if you locate a worthwhile class, you might be unable to find time for it as you work at a job or build a practice. Online courses have more flexible time requirements but, again, are not often on topic. Self-directed learning will be, if not your only option, at least your main option.

The cost of maintaining an educational program after your formal training has been completed is an important consideration. The effort requires you to invest both time and money, two commodities that may be in short supply, especially in the early stages of your career. Your motivation to improve your skills and the personal energy required to do so are also variables worth noting. You might feel you have put in enough educational effort and now would like to coast along on the results of that work. In counterbalance to that understandable inertia is the recognition that the more competent you feel, the more rewarding will be the hours you put into your job. In any case, most professions encourage, and sometimes require, documented continuing education to maintain your accreditation and licensure. Even if they do not recognize some of the educational tasks you undertake, such as keeping up with the literature or meeting with peers, the didactic return on those educational investments is reason enough to pursue them.

A helpful strategy is to set an educational budget at the beginning of each practice year, deciding in advance how much time and what level of funding you can afford to spend on this portion of your professional life. Expensed against this total would be the cost of conferences, books and journals, supervision, and other possible sources of continuing education. A realistic assessment of what moneys you can devote and of the time you can make available will allow you to manage both.

The Value of Experience

You will certainly benefit from the day-to-day practice of psychotherapy over time. Repetition in the exercise of the skills you have already acquired will improve your effectiveness. Exposure to a greater variety of clinical challenges will sharpen your abilities and present opportunities to employ your therapeutic tools against different problems. You will be a better therapist after a dozen patients and even more improved after 100.

Experience alone, however, is of limited value. It is unlikely to provide you with new abilities or to equip you with more effective techniques. In Figure 9–1, the bottom line shows a gradual increase in skills

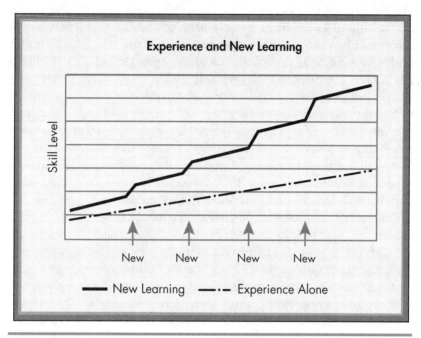

FIGURE 9–1. **Skill increase with new learning.**

over time. This line reflects the increase in existing skills if no additional learning takes place. The top line shows the effect of new learning. Each additional skill set elevates the curve and the level of overall competence.

If you are like most therapists, you will have left your training program wedded to one methodology. You will have been strongly influenced in this choice by the type of program you attended and, often, the methodology espoused by an admired faculty member or two. This selective beginning is useful. It is fair to say that it is a necessary choice. Concentration on a circumscribed area of practice allows maximum learning when time is limited. The choice of one methodology out of many reduces confusion and provides a sense of belonging. Inclusion in a particular "school" of psychotherapy is an important contribution to the formation of a professional identity, a development that usually occurs around the midpoint of your training.

Even though this phase of becoming a competent therapist is necessary, however, it is not sufficient to ensure the realization of your maximum potential in your field. If you do not continue to develop as a therapist, and instead remain committed only to whatever methodology you acquired in your training, you risk being only a one-trick pony.

The types of clinical problems you can effectively treat, and therefore also the number of patients you can help, will be limited by your single therapeutic approach. Although experience will improve your technical proficiency, the range of clinical presentations you can handle will not expand. Even as you master the single methodology you have chosen, you will become weaker in all the other skills to which you were introduced in training. In effect you will know more and more about less and less.

Another kind of experience—general life experience—is of great value to a therapist. You deal with a broad spectrum of socioeconomic life and with widely different aspects of the culture. Your patients will vary in level of education, ethnic background, occupational experience, and many other variables. The more you know about the society in which you practice, the more readily you will appreciate each patient's differing life circumstances and how they impact that patient's mental health. Activities and interests that expose you to the wider culture are a good source of learning about these differences. Culture is reflected in contemporary media and entertainment. The well-rounded therapist keeps up with the news, with online opinion, with popular television and published fiction, with sports, the arts, music, and politics. You may not agree with a patient's interests, values, political philosophy, or avocations, but the more familiar you are with the subject matter, the better you will understand your patients and the more easily you will empathize with their unique circumstances.

Also important in understanding your patients, and in understanding human nature in general, is an acquaintance with the recorded wisdom of those who were especially insightful about the subject. One set comprises the philosophers, psychologists, and social scientists who made significant contributions to our understanding of individual, family, group, and social behavior. Another set is the poets, playwrights, and novelists whose work gives a human face to the theories of the first. Reading widely in both areas will not only be rewarding in its own right but will pay dividends in your practice.

The Case for Technical Diversity

In Greek mythology Procrustes was an innkeeper on the road to Athens who offered travelers a pleasant meal and a night's lodging in his special iron bed. None of his lodgers would fit the bed exactly, so he would stretch the shorter guests on the rack and amputate the legs of the taller ones until all were the right length. The moral of this story for a therapist is that patients will be poorly served by a one-size-fits-all, single methodology treatment. A Procrustean approach will limit therapeutic success to only those patients whose needs exactly match the sole therapy on offer.

Even if you accepted that limitation—for example, if you only wanted to use a behavior therapy protocol to treat patients with panic disorder—human nature being what it is, you would still need additional skills. Your panic patients would develop transference feelings, so you would need some psychodynamic work. They might face existential problems or become depressed. In short, treatment failures with a single therapy approach would be high, and successful outcomes, even if narrowly defined, would be difficult to achieve. And how many of us would be happy with such a narrow, technical career?

Another way to limit what skills you need is to exclude a methodology. Suppose (as a trainee told me recently) you decided that cognitive-behavioral therapy was a boring, cookbook approach that stifled creativity (it isn't) and that you would refuse to use it. Faced with an appropriate patient—someone with dysthymia, for instance—you could refer them elsewhere or treat the problem with a different type of therapy. In the first case, you would lose a patient and perhaps annoy a referral source, who would look elsewhere the next time. In the second case, your alternative treatment might be less effective, a disservice to the patient and (unless you did not care about results) unsatisfactory for you.

Some therapists solve this problem by a combination of methodologies. Over time they develop a personal admixture of exploratory, directive, and experiential techniques into a single, idiosyncratic approach. With each patient they might deal with some material in an interpretive mode, cognitively challenge other material, and reflect the patient on other subjects. They have, in effect, created a single, all-purpose methodology out of these selections, a personal style, that they can apply to every patient. This blending of methods is likely to suffer some of the same drawbacks as the single "school" of psychotherapy, since their work is still somewhat limited, less creative, and, well, Procrustean.

A possible solution to this challenge may be an eclectic approach (Figure 9–2). Here you would develop a core group of methodologies with which you were most familiar and had the strongest skill set. The two or three or four therapies in this core group would allow you to deal with a majority of the patients who sought your help. The *core therapies* might include cognitive and psychodynamic therapies; at least, those two seem to have the widest application at present. Another set of skills, the *adjunctive therapies,* would comprise methods that would help you with patients who presented with unusual problems. For example, you

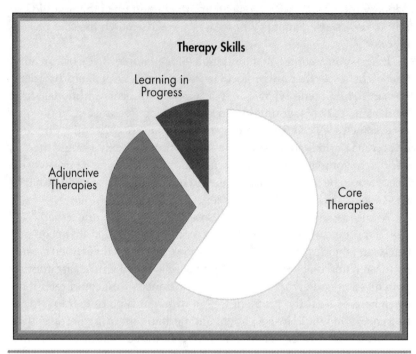

FIGURE 9–2. Therapy skill sets.

could employ hypnosis for a patient with dissociative identity disorder or posttraumatic stress disorder. The final group would include therapies you plan to develop into core or adjunctive strategies but did not yet consider yourself skilled enough to bring into regular use. These methods would be "learning in progress." Perhaps here you would have psychodrama or gestalt therapy, modalities that you might have encountered in your reading.

Self-Directed Learning

Fortunately, several avenues of posttraining education are available (Table 9–1). Some require out-of-pocket payment, and others are essentially free, costing only an investment of time. Unlike a training program, the decision about what to study, when to do so, and whether the investment is worthwhile is entirely up to you. You can think of the following discussion of self-directed learning opportunities as falling into two categories: passive and active learning. In the passive group are those experiences in which you are the recipient of knowledge offered by experienced and expert practitioners. Formal courses, books, and periodicals are in this category. Active learning includes the various supervisory and hands-on pursuits described below. While both types of learning can be useful, active participation is more likely to result in the acquisition of new and better skills and methods.

Formal Education

Formal coursework varies from a two-hour seminar to yearlong courses. Many supply a certificate of completion that is useful for documenting continuing education requirements for professional licensure or accreditation. The qualifications of those who offer them are usually vetted by reputable institutions or professional societies. The course content, however, may not offer the type of information and instruction you need to raise your therapeutic proficiency or acquire new techniques. Psychotherapy does not seem to be a popular topic of instruction. It is as if everyone assumed you were already competent in it. Quality programs in psychotherapy are uncommon. Even when you do enroll in one, it is not unusual to find only one or two useful new ideas in several hours of participation in one of these classrooms.

- Online courses ("distance learning") are often oriented toward specific situations or patient groups rather than skill sets. They are sometimes sponsored by marginal organizations. They can be costly. It is difficult to assess their value.
- Courses given by reputable institutions are usually site-based. The Beck Institute (cognitive therapy) is in Philadelphia. The Institute for Psychoanalytic Education (psychodynamic psychotherapy) is in New York City. Unless you are based in the city where the course is located, time and distance become problems. These programs are expensive.
- Continuing education (CE) courses may be sponsored by a particular professional association for their accredited members. The courses are often narrowly focused and unrelated to psychotherapy. Tuition fees can be nominal.
- Seminars and courses given at professional meetings, like CE courses, may not be relevant and require time and travel. Both the meeting and the courses can be high-priced.

TABLE 9–1. Educational resources

Resource	Availability	Monetary cost	Time investment	Convenience	Quality	Relevance
Formal training	Local	High	High	Low	High	Limited
Online courses	Limited	Low to moderate	Moderate	Moderate	Low	Moderate to high
Continuing education	Limited	Variable	Low to moderate	High	Moderate	Limited
Published resources	High	Moderate	Moderate	High	Moderate to high	Moderate to high
Individual supervision	Local	Moderate	Moderate to high	High	Variable	High
Peer supervision	Local	Low	Moderate to high	High	Variable	High
Single case exercise	Local	Low	High	High	High	High

Published Resources

A vast library of published material, like a dense forest spread out in all directions, is available in both periodical and book form, not only on the general topic of psychotherapy but also on innumerable narrow and specialized subjects.[1] How to find, in this dark wood, the few trees you need is a challenge. Because of their limited market, the cost of these published materials tends to be high. They can be worth the investment of reading time and of money, but selective judgment is needed to find the material you want. A journal might have only one or two articles of interest. A book could offer only a relevant chapter or two.

Journals

- *American Journal of Psychotherapy*
- *British Journal of Psychotherapy*
- *Journal of Contemporary Psychotherapy*
- *Journal of Psychotherapy Integration*
- *Psychotherapy*
- *Psychology and Psychotherapy: Theory, Research and Practice*

Publishers

- American Psychiatric Association Publishing
- APA (American Psychological Association) Books
- Guilford Press
- Jason Aronson Books (Rowman & Littlefield)
- Springer Publishing Company

Supervision

One-on-one and small-group instruction are the most efficient kinds of learning environments. Since the topics and subject matter are set by the participants, the relevance of the discussions is high. The investment of

---

[1] A recent enhancement is the addition of instructional video, either embedded into or accompanying printed and online material, that explains particular strategies and techniques. A variety of online psychotherapy demonstrations are now available as video on optical media or streamed. See, for example, psychotherapy.net and various postings on youtube.com.

time and money is variable but can be quite manageable on a modest educational budget. These pursuits are all carried out locally, without extensive travel, and can be programmed in manageable time allotments and on a convenient schedule.

Individual supervision is a well-recognized and respected learning strategy. No doubt you spent a significant portion of your professional training benefiting from this type of instruction. Once you are launched on your career, however, private supervision may be hard to come by. Psychotherapists who would be excellent supervisors may be busy with their own career responsibilities and unable to devote the time to this "extracurricular activity." If you can find a supervisor whom you respect or you know by reputation, and who is willing to work with you, act accordingly. As Polonius says to his son,

> Those friends thou hast, and their adoption tried
> Grapple them to thy soul with hoops of steel.

The supervisor would likely have his or her own ideas about how to structure the experience, but some routes to consider are to:

- Get help with formulating your cases and constructing an appropriate treatment plan, assistance that might avoid an impasse or other treatment problems later on.
- Follow one or two ongoing cases, which is often the best use of supervisory time.
- Troubleshoot problem cases as they come up.
- Provide instruction in a particular methodology.

Peer supervision is perhaps the least expensive and most convenient educational enterprise of all. You and some number of your peers—anywhere from two to six is reasonable—meet on a regular schedule to discuss cases and whatever topics they generate. It is a flexible undertaking. Groups can

- Discuss a single case at each meeting.
- Share progress on individual cases in roundtable fashion.
- Rotate case presentations on a weekly or less frequent basis.
- Review a journal article on a relevant topic.
- Present a brief summary of a topic of mutual interest.
- Troubleshoot problem cases.
- Discuss clinical and other practice problems.
- Consider current events that impact therapy practice.

Peer supervision has its drawbacks as well.

- Depending on the make-up of the group, a less experienced set of peers may not be as helpful as those with better developed skills. It could be a case of "the blind leading the blind."
- Stability of the membership, an important factor in developing comfort, confidence, and coherence in the group, may be undermined by changes in the status or external circumstances of the members.
- Interpersonal dynamics may impact the smooth functioning of the group and distract from the task.
- Without clear leadership or an agreed-on format, the discussion can deteriorate into unproductive channels or trivial topics, such as pointless discussions of therapy tactics.

A special instance of peer supervision that can be especially helpful is to follow one case under direct observation. Perhaps you had the opportunity in training to observe a supervisor or a colleague conduct therapy with a one-way screen set-up or a video recording of an ongoing case. This valuable experience can be duplicated, although with some difficulty, as part of a peer group experience. You probably do not have access to a one-way observation set-up, so you would have to opt for the video version. This approach increases the time commitment and can create its own difficulties.

- The exercise requires a confident therapist who is willing to be observed by others.
- The observation itself can distort the therapy process, although not as much as you might expect, since the observers are often ignored by both participants after the initial novelty wears off.
- Patient selection can be difficult.
- Audio recordings are far less useful than video because the observers lose all of the nonverbal information and thus miss an important part of the interactions.

Yet another way to follow a case in this manner, although it omits the benefit of direct observation, is to have one of the members volunteer to make a detailed record of each session and then present the result to the group.

- These process notes should contain relevant facts but not, obviously, every word the patient says.

- Patient narratives can be summarized to save time, but any direct therapeutic interaction between therapist and patient should be described to the group.
- Oddly, the greatest benefit may accrue to the therapist who treats the patient. The exercise of making a detailed report of your actions and ideas can be instructive. It can expand your thinking about the case and about how you conduct therapy in general.

Solo Learning

Useful learning can take place even without the instructive efforts of others. Sitting with patients presents many opportunities to improve your existing skills and to develop new ones.

Some of your new learning will take place without any special effort on your part. You do not always need to go elsewhere and spend additional funds on your continuing education, important as these avenues may be. As you conduct a therapy with each new patient, some things will work and others will not. These experiences will modify your therapy skills and shape your overall behavior. This trial-and-error learning will have a greater influence early on, but, given the complexity of this endeavor, such learning will continue to operate throughout your career.

You will encounter from your reading and from discussion with others new ideas and possible techniques that you can incorporate into your own practice. In my medical training days, we used to have a saying: "See one, do one, teach one." It reflected the magnitude of expected new learning—diagnostics, procedures, treatments—and the relative shortage of time to learn them. You observed, you tried it out, you helped your colleagues to learn it.[2] The process of modeling our behavior after those we watched and our partial identifications with them helped us overcome our trepidation about trying new things. In the same spirit, you can try out new things in your clinical work without the benefit of direct instruction. You are likely to be successful because

- You have a talent for therapy work, otherwise you would be in some other field.
- You will be building the new strategies and tactics on the foundation of your existing skills.

---

[2]Our anxiety about this truncated practice was reflected in our joking rearrangements of the sequence: "Teach one, do one, see one."

- Your therapeutic alliance will make the successful addition of the new approach easier for the patient to accept and profit from.
- Trial-and-error learning and modeling will help you modify any snags in the new process.

Final Thoughts

The emphasis in a formal course is on the content of the lecture: the history, theoretical underpinnings, instructions, and explanations that are transmitted in a classroom format from the instructor to the student. Of at least equal importance, however, is the manner and style demonstrated in the process of instruction:

- How the relationship is managed
- How the therapist sits, behaves, and speaks
- What kind of diction is used
- What response the therapist has to the emotions and actions of the patient

All of this information, although not part of the factual data, is important to absorb. Learning by modeling and partial identification is the result of exposure to this kind of information. In the various educational modalities I have mentioned in this chapter, supervision and the direct observation of therapy provide the best opportunities for this important learning process. In deciding how to structure your self-directed learning, you should look especially for these valuable opportunities.

Key Points

- After you complete your formal training, the onus of further professional development requires ongoing, self-directed learning.
- You will improve with experience, but the increase in your skills will be significantly greater if you continue to pursue new learning opportunities.
- The greater your technical diversity, the more effective you will be in practice and the better the outcome for your patients.
- Self-directed learning may include
  ➢ Formal coursework and published resources.
  ➢ Individual or peer group supervision.
  ➢ Solo learning.

CHAPTER TEN

What Is the Sum and Substance?

Change is the business of psychotherapy, and therapeutic change must be expressed in action—not in knowing, intending, or dreaming.

Irvin D. Yalom

Never answer an anonymous letter.

Yogi Berra

Summary

The preceding chapters have described the general characteristics of that curious activity known as psychotherapy. Therapist and patient, meeting on a regular schedule, undertake the collaborative task of improving the patient's mental and emotional condition. Only a persistent change in the patient's dysfunctional behavior can qualify as a psychotherapeutic improvement.

- Psychotherapy has a long tradition in the human saga. Its roots stretch back into tribal prehistory. Our modern brains respond to the same forces and influences as did our ancient ancestors'. Many of psychotherapy's attributes are shared by religious, supernatural, commercial, and political activities.
- Our contemporary version has developed over a period of two centuries, and its practice has splintered into hundreds of separate methodologies.
- Society sanctions psychotherapy and provides it with some basic protections, but still views it with a mixture of acceptance and suspicion.

305

- The corporate takeover of healthcare has burdened it with rules and restrictions. The legal system has added its own hazards. Government regulation has further constrained healthcare. In spite of these formidable headwinds, psychotherapy has continued to offer a valuable and increasingly more accessible benefit.

Psychotherapy is an activity hard to define in absolute terms. A variety of services available to those seeking help with psychological problems share some of its characteristics. In its most general sense, however, it seems to be a transactional process designed to bring about behavioral change within an asymmetrical power relationship. This book has examined the factors involved in dyadic therapy and provided by someone with the professional training to be called a psychotherapist.

The relationship between the two participants has three components:

- The *real relationship* is the nontherapeutic portion—the administrative and undistorted association required for the business of the activity.
- The *therapeutic alliance* is a mixture of personal and professional connections that develops between the participants and fuels the entire healing enterprise.
- The *operational plan* is the result of employing one or more methodologies in pursuit of a set of treatment goals that together will produce the desired outcome of the work.

Of the three components, the therapeutic alliance is the indispensable factor, the rate-limiting step, the sine qua non that determines therapeutic success. At its core, therapy is an effort at persuasion, based almost entirely on an indirect approach, and its effectiveness depends on the strength of the alliance. Because of the central importance of the alliance, a therapist should make every effort to strengthen and sustain its effects. To do so a therapist must

- Provide a safe, inviting, confidential, and professional environment.
- Demonstrate warmth, empathy, concern, respect, due care, and unconditional positive regard.
- Accept and utilize the emotional disposition and the recuperative impulses displayed by the patient.
- Maintain focus on the desired outcome, whatever distractions and resistances may arise.

The therapeutic alliance begins with an initial evaluation, one or more meetings designed to

- Establish a diagnosis.
- Illuminate the nature and importance of the patient's psychological problems.
- Develop a coherent explanation for those problems, a formulation.
- Determine what the patient wants and what the therapist is willing and able to provide: a treatment plan.
- Negotiate an agreement on what the two will attempt to achieve.

Once under way, the therapeutic alliance supports and energizes the chosen methodology. The work of any therapy is beset by problems that usually arise from difficulties with the communicative process and from counterforces to collaboration. These problems may weaken or even rupture the alliance, which remains a necessary concern of the therapist, who must suspend the operational plan in order to repair and rebuild it.

A therapist should be committed to professional development through self-directed learning.

The Career of a Psychotherapist

The profession of psychotherapy is a subcategory of several healthcare occupations. Psychiatry, psychology, and social work are the three most common careers, but nursing, physician assistants, and a variety of counseling specialties are a significant segment of the psychotherapy community. The discipline of psychotherapy usually requires a long period of preparation with a costly investment in formal education, supervised experience, certification, and licensure. Its practice provides both frustrations and satisfactions. Among the frustrations:

- Much of the time you deal with chronic illness.
- Patients' improvement is often slow and uncertain.
- You encounter difficult, sometimes vexatious, individuals.
- Those you try to help seem to oppose every effort you make.
- The work is labor intensive and emotionally wearing.
- The lack of a scientific basis makes it hard to know what are the best methods.
- Healthcare corporations and government agencies impose restrictions.
- It is not a pathway to wealth and fame.

The satisfactions include:

- The opportunity for an intimate understanding of other people's lives.
- The intellectual challenge of unraveling complex patterns of behavior.
- The emotional rewards of gratifying, valued work.
- The satisfaction of using interpersonal and persuasive skills for meaningful purposes.
- The ability to help people improve through significant behavioral changes.
- The prospect to make a decent living through reputable work.
- The possibility of being your own boss.
- The social status of participation in one of the healing professions.

The outcome of therapeutic work depends more on the character of the therapist than on the utility of any specific treatment method. It is perhaps fair to say that if you are the right person for this work, you will be successful whatever school of psychotherapy you espouse and regardless of your specific technical expertise. If you have the personality and the passion, your patients will benefit from their contact with you. Their lives will be better and, as the agent of therapeutic change, so will yours. The sum of these factors suggests that the choice of psychotherapy as an occupation is more of a calling than a job. It requires both diligence and dedication and would seem to favor those with compassion, empathy, creativity, verbal fluency, and emotional intelligence. If you are that kind of person, your way seems clear.

Or, as Yogi Berra advised: When you come to a fork in the road, take it.

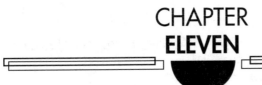

CHAPTER
ELEVEN

Suggested Readings

Be not the first by whom the new are tried,
Nor yet the last to lay the old aside.

Alexander Pope

I'm not going to buy my kids an encyclopedia. Let them walk to school like I did.

Yogi Berra

The literature on psychotherapy, both periodicals and published books, constitutes an enormous repository of research, theory, clinical material, methodology, and process. It is too much for any one person to read and assimilate. Since the field is fluid and fashions change rapidly, some of this written material seems contradictory and, at times, argumentative. Lacking the scientific basis of medicine and the "hard" sciences, whose theories nevertheless change from time to time as new findings emerge or old beliefs prove incorrect, psychotherapy texts often read more like a set of convictions than an exposition of facts.

The books listed here are, therefore, simply a set of personal preferences: a few books that might be useful as a foundation for the study of psychotherapy. This listing is in no way meant to be complete or, conversely, to suggest that other books may not be equally useful. The list includes histories and works of theoretical importance, because a therapist should appreciate the background and the antecedents of what we do today. The books on methodology and strategy are representative works on a few main topics or are related to topics covered in the preceding chapters.

History

A History of Medical Psychology, by Gregory Zilboorg and George W. Henry. New York, W.W. Norton, 1941.
From prehistory to the end of the Freudian era.

History of Psychotherapy: Continuity and Change, Second Edition, edited by John C. Norcross, Gary R. VandenBos, and Donald K. Freedheim. Washington, D.C., American Psychological Association, 2011.
Modern psychotherapy.

The Discovery of the Unconscious: The History and Evolution of Dynamic Psychiatry, by H.F. Ellenberger. New York, Basic Books, 1970.
A close examination of dynamic ideas.

Theory

The Ego and the Mechanisms of Defense, Revised Edition, by Anna Freud. Madison, Connecticut, International Universities Press, 1966.
The psychoanalytic mechanisms of common psychological processes.

Persuasion and Healing: A Comparative Study of Psychotherapy, Third Edition, by Jerome D. Frank and Julia B. Frank. Baltimore, Maryland, The Johns Hopkins University Press, 1991.
The seminal study of why psychotherapy "works."

Identity and the Life Cycle, by Erik H. Erikson. Psychological Issues 1:1. New York, International Universities Press, 1959.
Dynamic developmental theory.

Cognitive Therapy and the Emotional Disorders, by Aaron T. Beck. New York, Meridian, 1979.
The original ideas of the founder of this approach.

Personality and Psychotherapy: An Analysis in Terms of Learning, Thinking and Culture, by John Dollard and Neal E. Miller. New York, McGraw-Hill, 1950.
The authors combined psychoanalytic ideas with learning theory to propose a new, social learning theory.

Formulation as a Basis for Planning Psychotherapy, by Mardi J. Horowitz. Washington, D.C., American Psychiatric Press, 1997.
A practical example of traditional formulation and planning.

The Mask of Sanity, by Hervey Cleckley. New York, The New American Library, 1982.
   The classic study of the psychopath.

Treatment Planning for Psychotherapists: A Practical Guide to Better Outcomes, Third Edition, by Richard B. Makover. Arlington, Virginia, American Psychiatric Association Publishing, 2016.
   The case for treatment planning and how to do it.

Methodology

Transactional Analysis in Psychotherapy: A Systematic Individual and Social Psychiatry, by Eric Berne. New York, Grove Press, 1961. See also: **Games People Play: The Psychology of Human Relationships**, by Eric Berne. New York, Grove Press, 1964.
   An original theory of interpersonal psychology. Games People Play *was a bestseller.*

Existential Psychotherapy, by Irvin D. Yalom. New York, Basic Books, 1980.
   A comprehensive overview of the field.

The Technique and Practice of Psychoanalysis, Volume 1, by Ralph R. Greenson. New York, International Universities Press, 1967.
   One of the best explanations of this topic. He never wrote a second volume.

Concise Guide to Psychodynamic Psychotherapy, Third Edition, by Robert J. Ursano, Stephen M. Sonnenberg, and Susan G. Lazar. Washington, D.C., American Psychiatric Publishing, 2004.
   A useful overview.

Cognitive Behavior Therapy, Basics and Beyond, Second Edition, by Judith S. Beck. New York, Guilford, 2011.
   An example of a "how to" handbook.

Strategy

Strategies of Psychotherapy, Second Edition, by Jay Haley. Rockville, Maryland, The Triangle Press, 1990.
   A communications engineer by training, Haley made many original contributions.

Differential Therapeutics in Psychiatry: The Art and Science of Treatment Selection, by Allen Frances, John Clarkin, and Samuel Perry. New York, Brunner/Mazel, 1984.
   A guide to the eclectic approach to multiple methodologies.

General Interest

Learned Optimism: How to Change Your Mind and Your Life, by Martin E. P. Seligman. New York, Vintage Books, 2006.
> *A popular "how-to" book based on the author's (and others') research into "learned helplessness."*

Passages: Predictable Crises of Adult Life, by Gail Sheehy. New York, E. F. Dutton, 1976.
> *A lay reporter's review of developmental research. A best-seller in its day.*

Thinking Fast and Slow, by Daniel Kahneman. New York, Farrar, Straus & Giroux, 2011.
> *An important contribution to understanding how we (and our patient's) think.*

The Social Conquest of Earth, by Edward O. Wilson. New York, Liveright Publishing Company, 2012.
> *An original thinker explains why we are the dominant species.*

Index

*Page numbers printed in **boldface** type refer to tables or figures. Page numbers followed by n refer to notes.*